'Magnetoencephalography (   ) to
provide new insights into bra   ease,
providing a richness of infor   any
other non-invasive techniqu   xity
means that MEG can be dau   hers.
In this book, Dr Perry provides an excellent introduction to the core
physical principles underlying MEG, the nature of the data and the
questions that can be asked, before covering the different approaches
to source localisation and analysis. The book is therefore highly
recommended for anyone interested in either starting to use MEG
in their own research or simply learning more about this powerful
tool for neuroscience research.'

Krish Singh, Cardiff University

'The reader is taken on the journey from experimental conception to
data interpretation, this exceptionally useful and accessible resource
will be invaluable to researchers starting out in MEG.'

Matthew Brookes, University of Nottingham

Working with MEG

Working with MEG provides an accessible, user-friendly guide to using magnetoencephalography (MEG) in neuroscience research.

In this novel guide, Gavin Perry delves into the practical aspects of designing, running and analysing MEG studies – which have traditionally been transferred informally by lab support or word of mouth from more experienced researchers, a difficult and time-consuming task. This user-friendly guide provides those starting out in MEG research with these basics, giving them an understanding of concepts and terminology, guidance on using equipment as well as an overview of the strengths and limitations of the technique. The book is packed with example figures and contains a glossary of key terms. Chapters in this book cover topics such as the physiological origins of the brain's magnetic field, MEG instrumentation and how it can be used to measure brain activity, the process of collecting MEG data and how to design experimental paradigms for use with MEG. It also examines the fundamentals of MEG data analysis, including analysis in the time, frequency and time–frequency domains; performing analysis of the sources of the MEG signals within the brain; and using statistical methods to perform hypothesis testing on MEG data, as well as examples of some of the most commonly used applications of MEG.

Designed to be a practical guide for those new to the use of MEG as a research tool, this book will be essential reading for undergraduate, postgraduate and early career researchers looking for an introduction to MEG.

Gavin Perry is Multimodal Laboratories Manager at Cardiff University Brain Research Imagine Centre (CUBRIC). His research interest is in the application of MEG to the study of visual perception.

Practical Guides to Neuroimaging

The Practical Guides to Neuroimaging series includes accessible and user-friendly guides to using neuroimaging in psychological research. Books in the series will help students gain a solid understanding of neuroimaging techniques and provide support to academics and practitioners in teaching these topics. Each book in the series outlines a history of the neuroimaging method, how to use the method, how to read the data and when the method should be used. Written by experienced authors and full of examples and images, these practical guides will be essential reading for those starting out in neuroimaging research.

Working with MEG: A Practical Guide to Magnetoencephalography
Gavin Perry

For more information about this series, please visit: www.routledge.com/our-products/book-series/PGN

Working with MEG

A Practical Guide to Magnetoencephalography

Gavin Perry

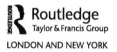

LONDON AND NEW YORK

Cover image: Maryna Ievdokimova/iStock via Getty Images

First published 2023
by Routledge
4 Park Square, Milton Park, Abingdon, Oxon OX14 4RN

and by Routledge
605 Third Avenue, New York, NY 10158

Routledge is an imprint of the Taylor & Francis Group, an informa business

British Library Cataloguing-in-Publication Data
A catalogue record for this book is available from the British Library

Library of Congress Cataloging-in-Publication Data
Names: Perry, Gavin, 1978– author.
Title: Working with MEG : a practical guide to
magnetoencephalography / Gavin Perry.
Description: Abingdon, Oxon ; New York, NY : Routledge, 2023. |
Series: Practical guides to neuroimaging |
Includes bibliographical references and index. |
Identifiers: LCCN 2022020380 (print) | LCCN 2022020381 (ebook) |
ISBN 9781138645080 (hardback) | ISBN 9781138645165 (paperback) |
ISBN 9781315205175 (ebook)
Subjects: LCSH: Magnetoencephalography.
Classification: LCC RC386.6.M36 P47 2023 (print) |
LCC RC386.6.M36 (ebook) | DDC 616.8/047548–dc23/eng/20220608
LC record available at https://lccn.loc.gov/2022020380
LC ebook record available at https://lccn.loc.gov/2022020381

ISBN: 9781138645080 (hbk)
ISBN: 9781138645165 (pbk)
ISBN: 9781315205175 (ebk)

DOI: 10.4324/9781315205175

Typeset in Bembo
by Newgen Publishing UK

To Joy Perry (1950–2021)

Contents

Preface

In 1968 at the University of Illinois, David Cohen made scientific history when he measured a neuronal oscillation known as the alpha rhythm from the brains of four human volunteers. The measurement of the alpha rhythm was not in itself a breakthrough: the German psychiatrist, Hans Berger, had discovered the rhythm decades earlier during his first recordings of human electroencephalography (EEG). What was novel about Cohen's experiment was that it did not measure electrical potentials on the scalp as is the case for EEG. Instead, the measurements were made using a metal coil built to measure magnetic fields. Cohen had become the first person to measure the brain's magnetic field and in doing so had pioneered an entirely new method for measuring the brain's activity: magnetoencephalograpy (MEG).

In the intervening decades MEG has grown from a highly specialised method practiced by a small number of researchers to a routine method of human neuroscience available at laboratories across the world. However, as the use of MEG has increased, so too has the number of people encountering MEG for the first time, and this has created a growing need for materials that aid the understanding of MEG for those with no prior experience.

When I first started working with MEG in 2006 there were few introductory guides to the technique. MEG was still a somewhat obscure methodology that you learned through a mixture of complicated technical papers heavy in mathematical equations, and informal lab wisdom passed on by word of mouth. Today there is a far greater range of articles and books offering an introduction to MEG (many of which are recommended in this book as further reading), but these often still tend to focus on the theory rather than the practical aspects of MEG and tend to assume some existing level of technical and mathematical knowledge on the part of the reader. Therefore, when I was invited to contribute this book to the Practical Guides to Neuroimaging series, I could see it would fill an important gap in the literature.

The purpose of the book is to serve as an introductory guide for researchers encountering (and using) MEG for the first time, explaining what MEG is, how MEG data can be acquired and how that data can be analysed and interpreted. I have not assumed any prior experience with MEG on the part of the reader (although I have assumed that the reader has some basic knowledge of human neuroscience). Because the book is intended as a practical guide aimed at beginners, I have also chosen not to include any mathematical equations, and instead to focus on qualitative rather than quantitative explanations of MEG. For those who wish to understand the mathematical details of the techniques described here (and anyone hoping to use MEG at an advanced level should be aiming to develop an understanding of the underlying mathematics) these can be found in many of the books and articles recommended as further reading at the end of each chapter. The focus of this work is on presenting the practical (rather than technical) details of MEG.

I am indebted to many people who have helped me complete this book. The series editor, Ceri McLardy, first proposed the idea of writing a practical guide to MEG – without that original idea and her ongoing support, this book would not have been created. I would also like to offer thanks to the rest of the editorial and production staff at Routledge, who have helped make this book a reality. My thanks go to Krish Singh for allowing me the time to work on this book and for useful comments and feedback on the book along the way. Diana Dima, Abi Finn, Eirini Messaritaki, Holly Rossiter and Rachael Stickland also provided feedback on draft chapters of the book, for which I am hugely grateful.

Finally, I would like to acknowledge the person who give this book existence by giving me existence: my mother. Sadly, she passed away during the writing of this book, but in life she was always supportive of my intellectual endeavours and would have been proud to see my work published. I dedicate this book to her.

Gavin Perry, April 2022

Figures

Part I

Measuring the brain's magnetic field

Chapter 1

What is MEG?

Magnetoencephalography (MEG for short) is the technique of measuring the brain's magnetic field. The idea that the brain produces a magnetic field is something people often find surprising: in everyday life we do not experience noticeable effects of magnetic attraction or repulsion around our heads. The reason for this is that the magnetic fields generated by the brain are extremely weak: too weak to be measured by all but the most sensitive of measurement devices. Indeed, it required the application of a type of highly sensitive magnetic sensor – known as a SQUID (short for Super Conducting QUantum Interference Device) – before the measurement of the brain's magnetic field became practical.

Given the difficulty of measuring the brain's weak magnetic fields, why does anyone go to the trouble of doing so? The reason is that there is a direct physical relationship between the electrical currents of the brain and the magnetic field measured outside the head, which means that (subject to limitations that we will explore as we progress though this chapter) MEG measurements give direct information about the brain's underlying electrical activity without requiring any invasive measurements. For this reason, MEG has emerged as an important tool for the measurement of brain function (and dysfunction) in humans.

The main strength of the technique is that, for all practical purposes, the magnetic field can be considered continuous in time, meaning that the rate of data acquisition is limited only by the rate at which the MEG hardware can operate. Commercially available MEG systems

DOI: 10.4324/9781315205175-2

can sample the magnetic field many thousands of times a second, meaning that data can be acquired at a sub-millisecond resolution. Thus, MEG can produce highly detailed information about changes in brain activity over time. Because the measurements can occur over a dense grid of locations across the surface of the head, MEG also provides information about the location of activity within the brain (albeit that it has poorer spatial resolution than some alternative techniques for localising brain activity such as fMRI). However, it is also true that there are many aspects of the brain's electrical activity that produce little or no magnetic field outside of the head. This means that not all aspects of brain activity can be measured with MEG. For those considering using MEG in their research or clinical practice it is therefore important to understand the kind of questions about brain activity that MEG can (and can't) answer, and to be aware of the strengths and weaknesses of the technique.

The purpose of this book is to act as an introductory guide to MEG for those starting out with the technique, and we will explore how MEG data is both acquired (Part I) and analysed (Part II). The aim of this first chapter is to help the reader to understand precisely what it is that MEG measures and how those measurements are made. We will start in Section 1.1 by describing how the brain's magnetic field is generated and what it can tell us about the underlying electrophysiological activity. Then in Section 1.2 we will look at the instrumentation used to perform measurements of the brain's magnetic field, in order to understand how those measurements are made.

1.1 What does MEG measure?

1.1.1 Introduction to magnetic fields

Magnetic fields occur whenever there is movement of electric charge. Therefore, every electric current acts as the source of a surrounding magnetic field, including the currents occurring within the brain. The magnetic field generated by an electric current extends into the surrounding space, and at each point in space the field has both a magnitude (measured in units of *tesla* [T]) and a direction.

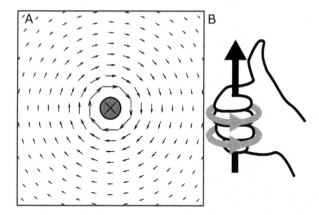

Figure 1.1 (A) Illustration of the magnetic field generated by current flowing away from the reader. (B) The 'right-hand rule' shows the direction of the field relative to the direction of the current.

Figure 1.1 A illustrates the magnetic field formed by a current flowing away from the reader into the page. The grey circle represents a cross-section of the wire through which the current flows and the length and direction of the surrounding arrows represent the magnitude and direction of the magnetic field at each point in the diagram. The direction of the magnetic field depends on the direction of the current and is given by the *right-hand rule* shown in Figure 1.1 B: when the direction of current (illustrated by the black arrow) is aligned with the outstretched thumb of the right hand, then the magnetic field (illustrated by the grey arrows) is oriented in the direction of the clenched fingers. The magnitude of the magnetic field is proportional to the strength of the current and, as can been seen in Figure 1.1 A, decreases with increasing distance from the current. In this illustration the field strength decreases proportionally to distance from the current (this corresponds to the field that would be generated by a theoretical current of infinite length).

Measurements of the magnetic field at different locations in space can therefore provide information about the strength, location and direction of the source current. This means that if we can measure the brain's magnetic field, then this should provide information about the strength, location and direction of electrophysiological currents occurring within the brain. This illustrates one of the reasons why the magnetic field outside the head is so weak: we are only able to measure the magnetic field at a relatively large distance from the source currents, where the strength of the field is much weaker than it would be if we could make measurements close to those currents, inside the head.

Because all electric currents generate a surrounding magnetic field, the magnetic field generated by the brain at each instant in time reflects the combined magnetic fields of all currents occurring within the brain. When two or more magnetic fields are present, the combined magnetic field depends on both the magnitude and direction of the individual fields. Where fields are oriented in the same direction they will combine constructively (i.e. they will add), but where they are in oriented in opposite directions they combine destructively (i.e. they will subtract). To illustrate this point, Figure 1.2 shows examples of the effects of two magnetic fields generated by pairs of wires with identical currents flowing in either the same or opposite directions. In Figure 1.2 A the two circles represent the cross-section of two wires in which current flows into the page (i.e.

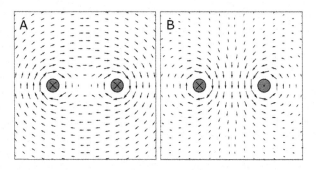

Figure 1.2 (A) The combined magnetic field generated by two currents flowing in the same direction (away from the reader). (B) The combined magnetic field generated by two currents flowing in opposite directions (the left current flows away from the reader, the right current towards the reader).

away from the reader), indicated by the two crosses. Figure 1.2 B shows the same spatial arrangement of currents but with the individual currents now flowing in opposite directions. The current in the right-hand wire now flows out of the page (i.e. towards the reader), indicated by the dot. In each plot, the combined magnetic field produced by the two currents is represented by the surrounding arrows.

By comparing the size and direction of the arrows at each location in the two plots, we can see that the strength and direction of the combined field differs depending on the spatial relationship between the currents that generate the field. When measuring the magnetic field at a distance from the source currents the field will be closer to that seen at the edges of each plot than towards the centre. As can be observed, the arrows tend to be larger – and therefore field tends to be stronger – at the edges of Figure 1.2 A (where the two currents flow in the same direction) than in Figure 1.2 B (where the currents flow in opposite directions). Thus, we can conclude that the magnetic field measured outside the head will tend to be stronger when the source currents flow in the same direction then when they flow in opposite directions. This conclusion will help to guide us as we look now at which currents contribute to the brain's magnetic field.

1.1.2 The magnetic field of a neuron

We have seen that magnetic fields are generated by electrical current, and that the brain's magnetic field is therefore a reflection of electric currents within the brain. But where exactly in the brain do these currents occur? To answer that question, we can start by looking at the electrophysiological currents occurring within individual neurons, and the magnetic fields associated with those currents.

The nervous system is a network through which information is processed and transmitted by the class of cells known as neurons. Each neuron can be thought of as both a processor and a transmitter in a complex network that coordinates cognition and behaviour. There are a multitude of varieties of neuron, but the majority have a common structure (Figure 1.3). Around the cell body – or *soma* – are a series of branching projections known as *dendrites* that form a

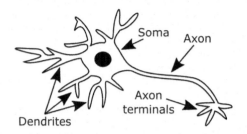

Figure 1.3 Diagram of a neuron illustrating its main structures.

complex, tree-like structure. Each neuron also has a long, thin projection – known as an *axon* – that extends outwards from the soma. The axon extends to one or more locations in the brain, where it separates into several projections – known as *terminals* – that each terminate close to the dendrites (or in some cases to the soma or axon) of another neuron. The membranes of the two cells do not touch but are separated by a narrow gap known as the *synapse*. Typically, each individual neuron has synapses with thousands of others.

The electrical properties of neurons are primarily due to ions present in the fluid medium that fills both the interior of the cell and the exterior space that surrounds the cell. The main ions involved are sodium, potassium, calcium (which are all positively charged) and chloride (which is negatively charged). The presence of these ions means that the fluid that fills the space both inside and outside neurons is electrically conductive, allowing electrical current to flow within the fluid. However, the ions cannot cross the cell membrane, meaning that the interior and exterior of the neuron are electrically insulated from one another. This isolation of ions on either side of the membrane is not complete, however, as distributed along the membrane are protein structures that allow specific ions to cross. The combined action of the various ion channels creates differences in the concentration of different ions in the interior and exterior of the neuron (particularly sodium, which has a higher concentration outside the cell, and potassium, which has a higher concentration inside the cell). Because these differences in concentration are not balanced, this leads to an excess of negative charge inside the cell (and positive charge outside the cell), and hence a difference in electrical potential (often known as a *voltage*) across the cell membrane, known as the *membrane potential*.

Many of these channels are *gated*, meaning that they open only under specific conditions. Some channels are voltage-gated, meaning that they only open when the difference in electrical potential across the cell membrane at their location is within a specific range. Others are ligand-gated, meaning that they open only when a specific signalling molecule – known as a *ligand* – is chemically bound to the channel. These gated channels, when opened, allow current to flow either into or out of the cell and this temporarily alters the membrane potential. Therefore, dependent on the current state of each of these gated channels, the membrane potential varies around the resting potential of the neuron.

At each synapse we can describe the cell that the axon extends from as being *presynaptic*, and the cell that the axon extends to as being *postsynaptic*. The presynaptic neuron can change the membrane potential of the postsynaptic neuron by releasing chemicals, known as *neurotransmitters*, that cross the synapses and bind to *receptors* on dendrites of the postsynaptic cell. This causes the opening of channels that allow ions move into or out of the cell. Because ions are charged particles, their movement across the cell membrane causes current to flow into or out of the postsynaptic cell. These currents produce localised changes in the electrical potential within the cell, known as *postsynaptic potentials* (or PSPs).

As shown in Figure 1.4, the postsynaptic potentials drive the flow of current within the dendrites (a representation of the time course of a postsynaptic potential at a location on the dendrite is shown in box A of Figure 1.4). This propagates changes in membrane potential around the cell, until the current 'leaks' out of the cell through channels that allow ions to cross back into to the extracellular space (the flow of current inside and outside of the cell is shown by the dashed lines in Figure 1.4). Currents that flow within the neuron as the result of postsynaptic potentials are often referred to as *impressed* or *primary* current. The impressed current is matched by current which flows in the opposite direction within the fluid medium outside the cell, known as *volume* or *secondary* current.

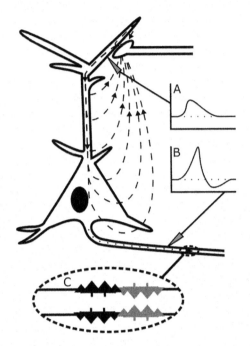

Figure 1.4 Illustration of neuronal currents and membrane potentials. Dashed line shows impressed and volume current generated by a postsynaptic potential (shown in box A). Dotted line shows the direction of propagation of the action potential (shown in box B). C shows a magnified representation of the axonal currents.

At any given instant, the neuron may contain a complex variety of postsynaptic potentials distributed throughout its interior that generate current flow both inside and outside the cell. Both the impressed and volume currents generate magnetic fields, and therefore measurement of the changing magnetic field over time can provide information about postsynaptic current occurring with in the neuron.

For the impressed current, the distances over which the current flows are much smaller than the distance from the neuron to the sensors at which the field is measured. Thus, when calculating the magnetic field generated by each current, we can treat the length of the current as negligible. The current can therefore be approximated by a theoretical current of infinitesimal length (i.e. the smallest possible length without being zero), known as a *current dipole*. A current dipole has no spatial extent (i.e. it is treated as occupying a single point in space) but has a direction (corresponding to the direction of current flow) and a magnitude (known as the dipole *moment* and measured in *ampere-metres* [Am]).

The magnetic field generated by a current dipole is the same as that shown in Figure 1.1 A, except that instead of decreasing in proportion to the distance from the current source, the strength of the field decreases in proportion to the *square* of the distance from the source. Thus, the field decreases even more steeply with distance than the field shown in Figure 1.1 A.

By contrast, the volume current flows throughout the entire volume of the extracellular space (and even the surrounding tissues) and therefore cannot be modelled by a simple point source such as a current dipole. To understand the magnetic field generated by volume currents it is instead necessary to model the geometry and electrical conductivity of the head. We will look at the effects of volume currents on the magnetic field outside of the head in Section 1.1.4.

Changes in electrical potential along the membrane and the dendrites are not the only source of electrical current within the cell. If changes in the membrane potential propagate to the axon and the potential drops below a level known as the *threshold potential*, this initiates an electrical impulse along the axon known as an *action potential* (a representation of the time course of an action potential at a location on the axon is shown in box B of Figure 1.4). When the initial segment of the axon reaches the threshold potential, this initiates the opening of voltage-gated sodium channels that allow current to flow into the cell (grey arrows in Figure 1.4 C) and causes a rapid depolarisation of the membrane, followed by the opening of voltage-gated potassium channels that allow current to flow out of the cell (black arrows in Figure 1.4 C) and cause a rapid repolarisation of the membrane. Thus, a burst of inward current flow followed immediately by a burst of outward current flow, causes a short-lived 'spike' in the membrane potential that propagates along the axon (shown by the dotted line in Figure 1.4). When the action potential reaches the synapses, it triggers the release of neurotransmitters that then alter the membrane potential of next the postsynaptic neuron. In this way, information is transmitted from neuron to neuron within the brain's neuronal network.

The currents of the action potential, like the postsynaptic currents, can be approximated as a point current source, because the distance over which the currents flow is negligible compared to the measurement distance. However, for most of the duration of the action potential there will be both an inward flow of current across the cell membrane and outward flow just slightly behind it along the axon (Figure 1.4 C). Thus, the currents associated with the action potential are like those shown in Figure 1.2 B, where two nearby currents flow in opposite directions. As we noted in the previous section, this arrangement of current produces a weaker magnetic field (when measured at a distance) compared to the field generated by currents oriented in the same direction. Therefore, in general we would expect the magnetic field generated outside the head by axonal currents to be weaker than the field generated by postsynaptic currents flowing within the dendrites.

More specially, if we treat the difference between the opposing currents flowing into and out of the axon as so small as to be negligible, the current can be modelled as a type of point source known as a *current quadrupole*. This is a source formed from two opposing currents of infinitesimal length separated by an infinitesimal distance (this can be visualised by imaging the opposing currents shown in Figure 1.2 B being brought as close together as possible). Whereas the strength of the magnetic field generated by a current dipole decreases with the square of distance from source, the strength of the field generated by a current quadrupole decreases in proportion to the *cube* of the distance. Thus, the field generated by the action potential decreases even more steeply with distance than that of the current dipole used to describe the postsynaptic currents and therefore will be much weaker when measured outside of the head. Additionally, the magnetic field must occur simultaneously across neurons in order to be measured outside the head (this will be explored further in the next section). Because action potentials are brief events lasting only a few milliseconds, this makes it less likely that they will overlap in time across neurons in order to produce a field strong enough to be measured outside of the head.

Due to these factors, it is therefore generally thought the currents generated by action potentials do not contribute significantly to the magnetic field outside of the head, except in rare circumstances in which neuronal firing is highly synchronised across a large population of neurons that are close to the MEG sensors. Instead, measurements of the magnetic field made outside of the head are believed to primarily reflect the postsynaptic currents flowing through the dendrites (and the associated volume currents) generated by postsynaptic potentials (Hämäläinen, Hari, Ilmoniemi, Knuutila, & Lounasmaa, 1993).

1.1.3 The magnetic field of populations of neurons

So far, we have seen that electrical currents generate a surrounding magnetic field, that this includes the electrical currents flowing in (and around) the neuron and that it is these currents that act as the source of the magnetic field that is measured with MEG. However, the currents generated by an individual neuron do not produce a strong enough magnetic field to be measured outside of the head. Only when the magnetic fields combine across many neurons does the field outside of the head become strong enough to be measured with MEG.

To understand the circumstances in which this happens, we first must note that postsynaptic currents flow longitudinally along the dendrites, and that their resulting magnetic fields are therefore oriented perpendicularly to the dendrites. This means that the contribution of each neuron to the magnetic field will be dependent on the spatial structure of its dendrites. For many types of neuron, the dendrites spread outwards from the soma in all directions, meaning that there is no tendency for the dendrites to be oriented in the same direction. As a result, there is also no general tendency for the magnetic fields generated by individual dendrites to be oriented in the same direction (Figure 1.5 A). Neurons with this property are

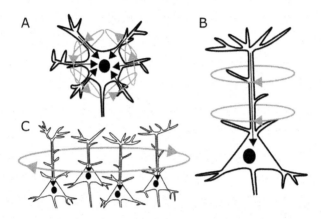

Figure 1.5 (A) A closed-field neuron in which the dendritic currents (black arrows) and the corresponding magnetic fields (grey arrows) do not tend to be oriented in the same direction. (B) An open-field neuron (a pyramidal cell) in which that dendritic currents and magnetic fields tend to have a single, dominant orientation. (C) The combined magnetic field across a group of pyramidal cells with synchronous currents.

known as *closed field* (Lorente de Nó, 1947). The magnetic field of these cells does not tend to combine strongly across dendrites (due to their differing orientations), and it is therefore possible for such neurons to produce little external magnetic field even when there is substantial impressed current within the dendrites.

Conversely, some neurons have dendrites that tend to be oriented in a specific direction relative to the soma, and hence have postsynaptic currents that tend to flow along that orientation. Such neurons are known as *open field* (Lorente de Nó, 1947). The most common type of neuron in the brain – the *pyramidal cell* – has dendrites with an open field structure. The soma of these cells has a distinct pyramid shape (hence their name) from the base of which extends both the axon and many short dendrites, known as *basal dendrites*. One or more relatively long dendrites – known as *apical dendrites* – extend from the apex of the pyramid. Because there are no long basal dendrites extending away from the soma in the opposite direction, the dendritic tree is asymmetric, and when current flows along the apical dendrite, a magnetic field is generated that is not cancelled by any opposing field in the opposite direction. The current flow within a pyramidal cell can thus be modelled as a current dipole oriented along the apical dendrites, with the corresponding magnetic field (Figure 1.5 B).

However, even where neurons have an open field structure, if the orientation of the dendrites varied across neurons, the magnetic field generated by each neuron would have a different direction and the fields would therefore tend to cancel. Fortunately, the apical dendrites of pyramidal cells in the cerebral cortex tend to be aligned perpendicularly to the surface of the cortex, meaning that current flow tends to have the same orientation across neurons within each small region of the cortex. This means that when current flows along the apical dendrites in the same direction, their magnetic fields combine rather than cancel (Figure 1.5 C).

For the fields to combine it is not only necessary for the currents to be spatially aligned but also to flow simultaneously in the same direction across neurons. Thus, electrical activity must be coordinated within a large, local population of neurons for there to be a measurable magnetic field outside of the head. One circumstance where this can happen is where a large population of neighbouring cells exhibit a simultaneous transient change in current: this leads to a corresponding transient change in the magnetic field. Such transient changes of the brain's magnetic field in response to an external event – such as the presentation of an external stimulus or the initiation of a behavioural response – constitute the event-related fields that are frequently the focus of MEG research (see Chapter 5).

Another scenario in which current flow can combine across neurons is where postsynaptic currents vary rhythmically. If these rhythms become synchronous across a large population of neurons the magnetic fields will combine, and this will cause the magnetic field outside the head to oscillate with the same rhythm (conversely, where the oscillations are asynchronous across neurons they will tend to cancel). These synchronous oscillations are another major component of the brain's magnetic that are often investigated using MEG (see Chapter 5).

Thus, while the magnetic field from a single neuron is too weak to be measured outside of the head, a sufficiently large number (tens or even hundreds of thousands) of open field neurons can produced a combined magnetic field strong enough to be measured outside of the head if they are in close proximity to each other and contain impressed current flowing synchronously in the same direction. In this case, the combined action of the currents flowing within the population of neurons can be treated as corresponding to a single current dipole, often known as an *equivalent current dipole* (Hämäläinen et al., 1993). The magnetic field outside of the head will depend only on the parameters that describe the position, orientation and moment of the dipole. The direction of the magnetic field around the population of neurons will follow the right-hand rule and the strength of the field will be proportional to the dipole moment (which is related to the total current within the population of neurons) and inversely proportional to the square of distance to the dipole (this means that the further the MEG sensors are from those currents, the weaker the magnetic field that will be measured by those sensors).

Where multiple local populations act as sources of the magnetic field, each can be treated as a separate dipole, and their contribution to the magnetic field outside the head can be approximated as the sum of the fields generated by each individual dipole.

1.1.4 The effect of volume current

In the previous section we have looked at how impressed current contributes to the magnetic field measured outside the head. However, as we observed in Section 1.1.2, postsynaptic potentials generate currents (known as secondary or volume currents) that flow outside of the neurons, and these currents also contribute to the brain's magnetic field. Thus, in order to understand the magnetic field generated outside the head by impressed current it is also necessary to take into account the contribution of volume current to the brain's magnetic field.

Because volume currents flow throughout the head, they generally cannot be characterised by point sources such as current dipoles, but instead must be calculated based on the shape and conductivity of the various tissues (such as the brain, skull and scalp) that make up the head. These can be modelled as a series of nested volumes each with a different shape and electrical conductance. For realistic models of the head, calculating the contribution of the volume current to the magnetic field involves complex mathematical modelling (we will look at some methods used for modelling volume currents when we look at solutions to the MEG forward problem in Chapter 4). However, a reasonable approximation can be achieved by modelling the head as a single spherical volume of homogenous conductance. In this case, the volume current does not need to be explicitly modelled, and instead the magnetic field outside of the head can be calculated from the parameters of the impressed current only (Sarvas, 1987). Specifically, in a volume of homogeneous conductance, the magnetic field outside the head depends on the degree of symmetry of the volume current around an axis defined by the impressed current (Grynszpan & Geselowitz, 1973): when the volume currents are perfectly symmetrical around the impressed current then no magnetic field is produced outside the head.

This symmetry occurs when a current dipole is oriented towards or away from the centre of the head (in this case the dipole is said to be *radially oriented*). As can be seen from Figure 1.6 A, a dipole with this orientation generates volume currents that are symmetric

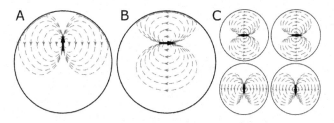

Figure 1.6 Illustration of impressed (black arrow) and volume current (grey dashed lines) for: (A) a radially oriented dipole; (B) a tangentially oriented dipole; (C) dipoles at the centre of the sphere.

around the dipole. The magnetic fields produced by the impressed and volume currents are exactly equal and opposite outside of the head, meaning that the two fields perfectly cancel. Conversely, where dipoles are at right angles to the radial orientation (and are therefore said to be *tangentially oriented*) the volume currents are not symmetrical, and the magnetic fields do not cancel (Figure 1.6 B). Thus, the magnetic field outside of the head is strongest for source currents oriented tangentially to the surface of the head and decreases as the orientation of the source approaches the radial axis. To the extent that the head is accurately modelled by a spherical conductor, impressed currents that have an exactly radial orientation produce no magnetic field outside of the head and therefore cannot be measured by MEG.

In the cerebral cortex, postsynaptic currents within the apical dendrites of pyramidal cells are oriented perpendicularly to the cortical surface, and therefore the corresponding equivalent current dipole is also oriented at rights angles to the cortical surface. Thus, MEG is generally most sensitive to currents flowing in parts of the cortex oriented perpendicular to the surface to the head (such as the two currents labelled A in Figure 1.7) and least sensitive to currents

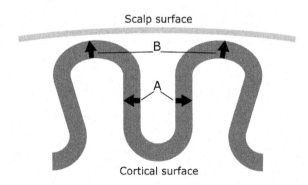

Scalp surface

Cortical surface

Figure 1.7 Illustration of the fact that source currents (shown by black arrows) can be (approximately) tangential (A) or radial (B) in orientation depending on the orientation of the corresponding area of the cortical surface.

flowing in parts of the cortex oriented parallel to the surface of the head (such as the two currents labelled B in Figure 1.7).

The symmetry of the volume currents around a current dipole is also influenced by the distance of the dipole from the centre of the sphere: the volume currents increase in symmetry as the distance of the dipole from the centre decreases. At the centre of the head the volume currents become perfectly symmetrical and therefore no magnetic field is produced outside the head regardless of the orientation of the dipole (Figure 1.6 C). Therefore, the magnetic field measured outside the head decreases with increasing depth of the source within the head.

Although the head is not a perfectly spherical and homogeneous conductor, this simplified model of the head gives a reasonable approximation of the effects of the volume current on the brain's magnetic field. The volume current modifies the magnetic field generated by sources of impressed current such that MEG is most sensitive to sources that are tangentially oriented and close to the surface of the head and is less sensitive to sources that are radially oriented and/or are at (or close to) the centre of the head (for a more detailed exploration of how the sensitivity of MEG varies across the cortical surface see Hillebrand & Barnes, 2002).

Before we end this section, we should also note that volume currents generate differences in electrical potential across the surface of the scalp. By placing electrodes on the scalp, it is possible to make measurements of differences in electrical potential in order to acquire information about electrophysiological activity occurring in the brain. This is the basis of electroencephalography (EEG), a technique closely related to MEG.

Because both techniques measure signals generated directly by the brain's electrical currents, MEG and EEG are closely related and can be used to address similar questions about brain activity. Both techniques share the property that measurements can be made at very high temporal resolution. The advantage of EEG over MEG is that sources at all orientations produce differences in electrical potential at the scalp, meaning that EEG is not blind to radial source currents. However, the spatial distribution of electrical potential across the scalp is distorted by the various tissues through which the volume currents pass (due to differences in their electrical conductance), meaning that more realistic (and therefore more complex) models of the head are necessary to estimate the location of the underlying source currents for EEG compared to MEG. Thus, while EEG measures more of the brain's electrical activity, it is easier to identify the source of the brain's activity using MEG. The techniques are not mutually exclusive, however, and MEG and EEG measurements can be acquired simultaneously. In theory, because the methods have different sensitivity to sources of different orientation, this provides greater information than can be provided by each technique in isolation (Cohen & Cuffin, 1983).

The use of EEG as a methodology is covered in a separate book in this series, but many of the analysis techniques described in Part II can be used with EEG as well as MEG.

1.1.5 Summary

We have seen that when electrical current flows through a conductor, a surrounding magnetic field is formed. Neuronal currents occurring in the brain generate a magnetic field and making measurements of this field – a technique known as magnetencephalography or MEG – can provide information about electrical activity in the brain. The MEG measurements primarily reflect postsynaptic currents flowing within neurons with an open-field structure, and their associated volume currents. In the cerebral cortex, this most likely corresponds to current flow within the apical dendrites of pyramidal cells. When there is synchronous current flow along these dendrites within a spatially aligned population of neurons, the combined magnetic field is strong enough to be measured outside the head. These currents can be modelled by one or more equivalent current dipoles and the magnetic field measured outside the head should closely correspond to the field produced by the corresponding dipole. However, the effect of volume currents means that MEG is not sensitive to neuronal currents at all positions and orientations within the head. Instead, sensitivity to dipolar sources becomes weaker as their orientation gets closer to the radial axis or their position gets closer to the centre of the head.

1.2 How is MEG measured?

So far, we have seen how the brain's magnetic field is generated and what information the field can provide about electrophysiological activity within the brain. In this section, we look at how the magnetic field is measured.

1.2.1 Measuring the brain's magnetic field

Making measurements of the brain's magnetic field is particularly challenging because the field is extremely weak when measured outside of the head. In Section 1.1.1 we have seen that the strength of the magnetic field is measured in units of tesla [T]. To give the magnitude of this unit some context: the strong static magnetic field produced by MRI scanners is usually in the range of 1.5–7 T; a typical fridge magnet has a field on the order of 10^{-3} T; while the Earth's magnetic field, measured at the surface, is on the order of 10^{-5} T. By contrast, the brain's external magnetic field is many orders of magnitude less than this and is generally measured in units of picotesla [pT] (10^{-12} T) or femtotesla [fT] (10^{-15} T). Thus, the magnetic fields measured using MEG are at least a billion times weaker than those of a fridge magnet!

This means that the sensors used to measure the brain's magnetic field must have extremely high sensitivity. For this reason, up until recently, all commercially available MEG systems measured the magnetic field using use a specific type of sensor known as a Superconducting QUantum Interference Device or *SQUID*. Superconductivity is a property of some materials that causes them to exhibit no resistance to electrical current when their temperature drops below a certain level, known as the *critical temperature* (sometimes denoted by T_c). The SQUID sensor is formed from a loop of superconducting wire around which an electrical current flows when exposed to a magnetic field. The loop contains a small gap known as a *Josephson junction*, which the current is able to cross due to an effect known as quantum tunnelling. This creates a difference in voltage across the gap which can be measured in order to quantify the strength of the magnetic field passing through the loop. These measurements can then be converted by electronic acquisition hardware into digital recordings of the magnetic field.

Because SQUIDs rely on superconductivity to operate, they must be cooled below their critical temperature to function. This is achieved by cooling them with liquid helium, which has a boiling point (-269 °C) that is below the critical temperature of the types of SQUIDs used for MEG. Because of this, the SQUIDs cannot be placed in direct contact with the head but are instead mounted within a thermally insulated helmet connected to a large vacuum container – known as a *dewar* – that holds the liquid helium. Unlike EEG, where measurements are made from electrodes that are attached to the subject's head at the required measurement locations, MEG SQUIDs are maintained in a fixed configuration within the MEG helmet and the subject is positioned with their head inside the helmet in order for data to be acquired.

In recent years, a new variety of sensor, known as an optically pumped magnetometer (OPM) has begun to be used as an alternative to SQUIDs. These sensors do not use superconductivity to measure magnetic fields (they instead measure the effects of the magnetic field on the atomic spin within a metallic vapour) and therefore do not have to be cryogenically cooled. This means the sensors can be attached to the subject's head, giving them two advantages over SQUIDs: the sensors are positioned closer to the scalp and therefore have greater sensitivity to the brain's magnetic fields and, because they are fixed to the subject's head, they are more tolerant of subject movement. At the time of writing, OPM-based MEG systems are beginning to become commercially available as an alternative to SQUID-based systems. Because SQUIDs are still the most widely used type of sensor for MEG, this book will assume that the reader is working with a SQUID-based MEG system. However, the principles of data acquisition and analysis described will also generally be valid for MEG research using OPMs.

When using SQUID-based sensors, the SQUIDs typically do not directly measure the magnetic field generated by the head. This is because the superconducting loop used to form each SQUID is typically small and therefore only measures the magnetic field over a small area. Instead, each SQUID is linked to a loop of superconducting

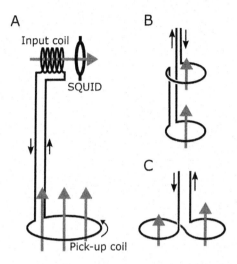

Figure 1.8 (A) Illustration of the circuit that forms a magnetometer. (B) The pickup coil configuration used for an axial gradiometer. (C) The pickup coil configuration used for a planar gradiometer.

wire known as a *pickup coil* that is positioned at the measurement location inside the helmet (Figure 1.8 A). The pickup coil is larger than the SQUID coil and therefore measures the magnetic field over a larger area. The current generated in the pickup coil is transmitted to a *signal coil* that is positioned close to the SQUID. The signal coil generates a magnetic field that is proportional in strength to the field measured by the pickup coil, meaning that the circuit containing the two coils transmit the magnetic field from the measurement location to the location of the SQUID (which is located deeper within the helmet). Importantly, as the signal coil is smaller than the pickup coil and contains multiple loops, the field is concentrated over a smaller area and hence the SQUID is exposed to a stronger field than if the external field was measured directly.

This arrangement also makes it possible to create SQUID-based sensors that measure different aspects of the magnetic field by using different arrangements of pickup coils. The simplest configuration for a MEG sensor involves each SQUID measuring the signal transmitted by a single pickup coil. In this case the SQUID acts as a *magnetometer*: a sensor that measures magnetic field strength. The SQUID measures the strength of the magnetic field in the direction perpendicular to the pickup loop (Figure 1.8 A).

An alternative arrangement that reduces sensitivity to environmental interference involves each SQUID being linked to two pickup coils that are wired in opposition. In this case currents flowing in the same direction in each loop oppose each other, and thus the signal measured by the SQUID is equal to the difference in the magnetic field between the loops, which can be interpreted as a measurement of the gradient of the field. Sensors configured in this way are known as *gradiometers*.

There are two types of gradiometer commonly used in MEG systems. In the first case the loops are placed in parallel, with one above the other (Figure 1.8 B). The SQUID then measures the gradient of the magnetic field in the direction perpendicular to the loops. A sensor with this configuration is known as an *axial gradiometer* (or less commonly as a *radial gradiometer*). In the second case the loops are placed side by side (Figure 1.8 C). Each loop measures the magnetic field in the direction perpendicular to the loop, but the SQUID measures the gradient of the field at a right angle to this direction. A sensor with this configuration is known as a *planar gradiometer*. Planar gradiometers normally come in pairs oriented at 90° from each other so that the field gradient can be measured in both directions within the plane of the pickup coils.

Because the gradient of magnetic fields decreases more rapidly with distance from the source than the strength of the field, gradiometers are less sensitive than magnetometers to more distant sources of magnetism. As most sources of magnetic interference are further from the sensor than the brain, this makes gradiometers less sensitive to interference. However, this comes at the disadvantage that gradiometers will also tend to be less sensitive to more distant brain sources than magnetometers. Some MEG manufacturers therefore include both magnetometers and gradiometers in their systems, so that the user can benefit from the different advantages of each type of sensor.

In theory, it is possible to combine two gradiometers in opposition to create a second-order gradiometer that measures the difference between the gradiometers, to create a third-order gradiometer by measuring the difference between a pair of second-order gradiometers, and so on. With increasing gradiometer order the sensors would become increasingly less sensitive to distant sources of magnetic noise. In practice, currently available MEG systems provide only first-order gradiometers, but some systems offer the possibility of synthesising higher-order gradiometers by measuring the difference in response between the primary sensors and a set of reference sensors.

Measurements from a single sensor gives the magnetic field (or field gradient) at one location (the location of the pickup coil). In order map the magnetic field across the surface of the head, MEG systems contain an array of SQUIDs connected to pickup coil(s) placed on the inside the helmet (Figure 1.9). The pickup coils form a dense array across the inner surface of the helmet in order to provide as much coverage of the head as possible. Each coil is aligned parallel to the surface of the helmet, meaning that each SQUID measures the component of the magnetic field perpendicular to the surface of the helmet.

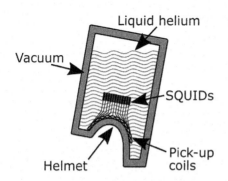

Figure 1.9 Layout of the key components in a typical SQUID-based MEG system.

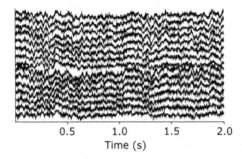

0.5   1.0   1.5   2.0
Time (s)

Figure 1.10 Example of raw data collected from a selection of 15 MEG sensors.

1.2.2 Sampling the magnetic field

For all practical purposes, we can consider the magnetic field around the head to be continuous in both space and time. In order to analyse the data using digital computers, it is necessary to record this continuous data as set of discrete data samples. It is these digitised time series of magnetic field measurements recorded from the array of sensors that forms the raw data of MEG (Figure 1.10).

The spatial aspect of this sampling process is determined by the spatial distribution of the MEG sensors. In designing the sensor array there is a fundamental trade-off: increasing the size of the coils produces a stronger signal but means fewer coils can fit inside the surface of the helmet leading to poorer spatial resolution. For commercially available systems this trade-off leads to sensor arrays that sample the magnetic field in the range of (approximately) one hundred to three hundred locations and have a spacing between sensors on the order of centimetres. It is this fixed spacing between the sensors that determines the spatial resolution of the data.

By contrast, the MEG sensors measure the magnetic field continuously in time, and do not impose any specific temporal resolution on the data. Instead, it is the process of converting these continuous measures into discrete samples (which is limited by the electronic hardware used to digitise the data rather than on the properties of the sensors) that determines the temporal resolution of the data.

The rate at which the continuous data is sampled is known as the *sampling rate* (and is measured in the unit of frequency: *Hertz [Hz]*). The time interval between data samples is the reciprocal of this rate (for instance, when data is acquired at a sampling rate of 500 Hz, the magnetic field would be sampled every 2 ms) and thus it is the sampling rate of the MEG system that determines the temporal resolution at which brain signals are measured. The sampling rate also places a fundamental limit on the measurement of periodic signals (that is, signals that periodically repeat, such as oscillatory brain responses), as these can only be measured for frequencies up to half the sampling rate. The maximum frequency that can be measured − corresponding to half the sampling rate − is known as the *Nyquist frequency*.

In practice, the temporal precision of the data will always be lower than would be theoretically expected by the sampling rate, due to an inherent problem in the process of sampling continuous signals, known as *aliasing*. To illustrate this problem, Figure 1.11 shows the process of sampling two periodic signals. The grey and black lines illustrate continuous signals at frequencies above and below the Nyquist frequency, respectively. The data points sampled from each

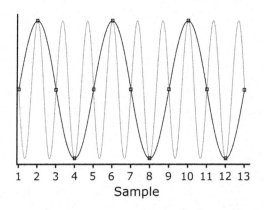

Figure 1.11 Illustration of the aliasing of a signal above the Nyquist frequency (grey line) with a corresponding signal below the Nyquist frequency (black line).

of the signals at each sampling interval – illustrated in the figure by white squares – are identical. Thus, the two signals are indistinguishable based on the sampled data, and the signal above the Nyquist frequency would be mistakenly measured as occurring at the corresponding frequency below the Nyquist frequency. Indeed, all signals at frequencies greater than the Nyquist frequency will be *aliased* to corresponding frequencies below the Nyquist frequency in the sampled data.

To prevent this problem, the acquisition electronics will apply a temporal filter (known as an *anti-aliasing filter*) that suppresses signals above a cut-off frequency before that data is sampled to remove signals above the Nyquist frequency (for more information about temporal filtering see Chapter 3). For periodic signals, the highest frequency that can be measured will therefore be determined by the cut-off frequency of the anti-aliasing filter. Because this filtering process is equivalent to smoothing the data in time, the precision with which brain signals can be measured in time will also be limited by the cut-off frequency of the filter.

In practice, sampling rates in the high hundreds or low thousands of Hz are typically used for MEG data acquisition, as this allows the cut-off frequency of the anti-aliasing filter to be greater than the frequencies of the brain signals (which mostly occur at frequencies below 100 Hz). The temporal resolution of the resulting MEG data may therefore be as low as fractions of a millisecond (although after anti-alias filtering the temporal precision of the data will more likely be on the order of milliseconds). While MEG data acquisition electronics can often support higher sampling rates than this, the size of the data increases proportionally to the sampling rate, and this leads to larger data sets that may be more difficult to store and process (particularly for data acquisitions of long duration).

1.2.3 Summary

In this section we have seen that the low strength of the brain's magnetic field means that, historically, only the most sensitive of magnetic sensors, known as SQUIDs, have been used to perform MEG. These superconductive sensors must be continuously bathed in liquid helium to function. Thus, rather than being directly mounted on the subject's head like EEG electrodes, the sensors are mounted as a fixed array inside a helmet attached to a large thermally insulated vessel that holds the helium. The SQUID-based sensors can measure either the strength (magnetometers) or gradient (gradiometers) of the component of the magnetic field perpendicular to the surface of the helmet.

More recently, a new type of sensor – the OPM – has also begun to be used to perform MEG. This sensor has some advantages over SQUID-based sensors, but for now most MEG measurements are still made using SQUIDs.

For the purposes of MEG, the magnetic field can be regarded as continuous in time and the rate at which measurements of the field can be made is limited only by the MEG electronics. It is this that leads to MEG having a high temporal resolution compared to other techniques, such as MRI. Commercially available MEG systems can support data acquisition at sub-millisecond temporal resolution (although in practice the temporal precision of the data will be less than this due to the need for anti-aliasing of the data).

Further reading

Baillet, S. (2017). Magnetoencephalography for brain electrophysiology and imaging. *Nature Neuroscience, 20*, 327–339. https://doi.org/10.1038/nn.4504

Buzsáki, G., Anastassiou, C. & Koch, C. (2012). The origin of extracellular fields and currents – EEG, ECoG, LFP and spikes. *Nature Reviews Neuroscience, 13*, 407–420. https://doi.org/10.1038/nrn3241

da Silva, F. H. L. (2010). Electrophysiological basis of MEG signals. In P. C. Hansen, M. L. Kringelbach, & R. Salmelin (Eds.), *MEG: An introduction to methods*, 1–23. Oxford University Press. https://doi.org/10.1093/acprof:oso/9780195307238.003.0001

Lee, Y. H., & Kim, K. (2014). Instrumentation for measuring MEG signals. In S. Supek & C. J. Aine (Eds.), *Magnetoencephalography: From signals to dynamic cortical networks*, 41–71. Springer. https://doi.org/10.1007/978-3-642-33045-2_1

Parkkonen, L. (2010). Instrumentation and data preprocessing. In P. C. Hansen, M. L. Kringelbach, & R. Salmelin (Eds.), *MEG: An introduction to methods*, 24–64. Oxford University Press. https://doi.org/10.1093/acp rof:oso/9780195307238.003.0002

Tierney, T.M. et al. (2019) Optically pumped magnetometers: From quantum origins to multi-channel magnetoencephalography. *NeuroImage, 199*, 598–608. https://doi.org/10.1016/j.neuroimage.2019.05.063

References

Cohen, D., & Cuffin, B. N. (1983). Demonstration of useful differences between magnetoencephalogram and electroencephalogram. *Electroencephalography and Clinical Neurophysiology, 56*(1), 38–51. https://doi.org/10.1016/0013-4694(83)90005-6

Grynszpan, F., & Geselowitz, D. B. (1973). Model studies of the magnetocardiogram. *Biophysical Journal, 13*(9), 911. https://doi.org/10.1016/S0006-3495(73)86034-5

Hämäläinen, M., Hari, R., Ilmoniemi, R. J., Knuutila, J., & Lounasmaa, O. V. (1993). Magnetoencephalography – theory, instrumentation, and applications to noninvasive studies of the working human brain. *Reviews of Modern Physics, 65*(2), 413. https://doi.org/10.1103/RevModPhys.65.413

Hillebrand, A., & Barnes, G. R. (2002). A quantitative assessment of the sensitivity of whole-head MEG to activity in the adult human cortex. *NeuroImage, 16*(3), 638–650. https://doi.org/10.1006/NIMG.2002.1102

Lorente de Nó, R. (1947). Action potential of the motoneurons of the hypoglossus nucleus. *Journal of Cellular and Comparative Physiology, 29*(3), 207–287. https://doi.org/10.1002/JCP.1030290303

Sarvas, J. (1987). Basic mathematical and electromagnetic concepts of the biomagnetic inverse problem. *Physics in Medicine and Biology, 32*(1), 11–22. https://doi.org/10.1088/0031-9155/32/1/004

Chapter 2

How to collect MEG data

Having established the origins of the brain's magnetic field and how it is measured, in this chapter we will explore in more detail the process of acquiring MEG data. In the first section of the chapter, we will look at the practical details of how MEG data is collected. This will be followed in the second section by an exploration of the design of experimental protocols for use with MEG.

2.1 MEG data acquisition

Compared to many other techniques, the process of acquiring MEG data is relatively straightforward: there are few safety issues, only a limited amount of participant preparation is required and there are few free acquisition parameters that need to be set. However, there are two keys issues that must be considered when collecting MEG data. Firstly, although MEG may have fewer safety issues than some other methods, it is not wholly risk free. To ensure that data is acquired safely users must be aware of these risks and the steps that can be taken to mitigate them. Secondly, because the MEG sensors are so sensitive, they are highly susceptible to interference from sources of magnetism other than the brain. Thus, is necessary to take steps to minimise these sources of interference to limit their effects on the data.

In this section we will give an overview of the procedures involved in MEG data acquisition, before giving a more detailed description of the safety issues involved, and of the sources of magnetism that

DOI: 10.4324/9781315205175-3

might interfere with measurements of the brain's magnetic field and the steps that can be taken to minimise them. We will end with an illustration of how MEG data can be acquired using a step-by-step workflow of a typical data acquisition.

2.1.1 Acquiring MEG data

A typical MEG data acquisition involves an individual experimental subject or patient being positioned with their head inside the MEG helmet (or in the case of OPM-MEG with the sensors attached to the head) so that their brain's magnetic field can be measured. These measurements can be made while the participant is at rest or while undergoing some form of sensory stimulation and/or behavioural task and are recorded as digital samples for subsequent analysis.

Figure 2.1 shows a schematic diagram of the basic layout of the hardware components used in routine acquisition of MEG data. One of the most notable elements of the MEG laboratory environment is that the MEG system is positioned inside a magnetically

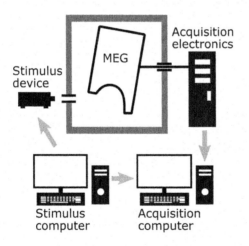

Figure 2.1 Schematic diagram of the main hardware components of the MEG laboratory. Grey arrows show the direction of communication between devices.

shielded room (MSR) that separates it from the MEG operator and the various computers and electronic equipment used in MEG data acquisition. This reflects the fact that the magnetic fields present in the laboratory environment are far stronger than the brain's magnetic field, and thus interfere with the MEG measurements.

The MEG sensors are connected to acquisition electronics located outside the shielded room via cables that pass through openings in the walls of the room. These openings are surrounded by metal cylinders called *waveguides* that restrict certain electromagnetic signals from entering through the opening and interfering with the magnetic field measurements made by the sensors. The electronics receive the measurements made by the sensors and convert them to digital samples. This information is then transmitted to a data acquisition computer that allows the operator to visualise the magnetic field measurements in real time and record the data to disk. The operator can also control features of the data acquisition such as which data channels (such as the sensors and other input devices connected to the system) to record, the duration and sampling rate of the acquisition and information about event triggers (see Section 2.2.3).

When working with SQUID-based MEG, each participant's head may be positioned differently within the helmet (and may also move during an acquisition) and so it is generally necessary to measure the position of the head relative to the sensors while performing data acquisition. This is achieved by attaching small electrical coils, known as *head localisation* or *head position indicator* coils, to the participant's head. These coils are connected to the MEG system, and, during data acquisition, each coil can emit a magnetic field that alternates at a set frequency. The signal from each coil can then be detected by the MEG sensors in order to measure the position of each coil within the helmet. This information is then used to record the participant's head position relative to the sensors in order to monitor and record the participant's head movement during the acquisition.

The MEG system will generally also incorporate hardware to perform electrophysiological recordings simultaneously with MEG data acquisition. These may be used as additional experimental measures or to aid with the identification of data artefacts occurring caused by physiological processes (see Section 2.1.3). This can allow the simultaneous measurement of EEG alongside MEG and can also be used to acquire other electrophysiological measures such as electro-oculography (EOG; the measurement of electrical activity due to movement of the eyes), electrocardiography (ECG; the measurement of the electrical activity of the heart) and electromyography (EMG; the measurement of electrical activity produced by the flexion or extension of muscle).

The set up described so far is all that is required to record MEG data while the subject is at rest. However, more commonly the user will wish to collect MEG data while the subject undergoes an experimental or clinical testing protocol involving some form of sensory stimulation and/or behavioural task. For this purpose, a second computer – referred to here as the stimulus computer – is used to interface and control the various stimulus and response devices. This computer will generally have one or more pieces of software for stimulus delivery and experimental control.

The MEG laboratory will have a variety of devices for different forms of sensory stimulation and behavioural response of the participant. All such devices ideally produce minimal magnetic interference to avoid introducing artefacts to the MEG data (see Section 2.1.3). Visual stimulation is usually generated by a projector positioned outside of the shielded room. Images are projected through a waveguide to a screen inside the shielded room positioned in view of the subject. Because conventional earphones and speakers contain magnetic components that will interfere with the MEG recordings, presentation of auditory stimuli is usually achieved by the transmission of sound along pneumatic tubes to specially designed foam buds placed in the participant's ear. MEG-compatible devices for generating other forms of sensory stimulation may also be available. Metal-free button boxes and other forms of non-magnetic response device that connect to the stimulus computer via fibre optic cables can be used for the measurement of behavioural responses.

The stimulus computer will have some form of connection to the MEG acquisition electronics, so that information about the timing of events (for instance, the onset of a stimulus or the timing of a response) can be recorded as part of the data. These normally are sent in the form of short duration digital inputs, sometimes called *triggers*, that mark the timing of experimental events and thus allow data to be analysed relative to the time of these events. Some stimulation and response devices may also have a direct connection to the MEG acquisition electronics so that outputs from these devices can also be used to mark event timing. We will look more closely at the design of experimental tasks and the use of event triggers in Section 2.2.3.

2.1.2 Safety

Because MEG does not involve ionising radiation or strong magnetic fields, it presents relatively few safety issues compared to other techniques, such as PET or MRI. However, although the risks are few, some can be highly dangerous (but thankfully also extremely rare). Therefore, before commencing with data acquisition, users must ensure that they understand correct safety procedures when working with MEG.

The biggest source of danger within the MEG laboratory is the presence of liquid helium within the MEG dewar. Although the helium is thermally insulated from the surrounding environment, this insulation does not completely prevent warming of the helium which slowly boils off over time. Under normal operating conditions the resulting gas escapes through an exhaust outlet (where it is either captured for reliquefaction or allowed to vent harmlessly into the atmosphere). If for any reason the helium gas was to leak into the shielded room instead, this would displace oxygen from the room and create a risk of asphyxiation for anyone present. This is particularly dangerous as helium has no odour or taste and does not produce the sensation of suffocation, so the asphyxiation might only become noticeable once the subject starts to lose consciousness.

Thankfully, incidences of helium leakage from a MEG system while in operation are extremely rare. However, because of the extremely high level of harm that may occur in such circumstances, all MEG laboratories will have systems and procedures in place to mitigate the risk posed by such an event. At the minimum, shielded rooms will be equipped with oxygen sensors that trigger an alarm when oxygen concentration in the room drops below a safe level. MEG users are therefore required to be familiar with this alarm (and any other signals that indicate reduced oxygen within the shielded room) and with local procedures on how to respond if the alarm is triggered.

In addition to the risk of asphyxiation, the low temperature of any leaked gas also presents a risk of harm. Leaked gas will have temperatures well below freezing and therefore direct contact with either the gas itself or surfaces that have been in recent contact with the gas can lead to cold burns. Any signs of visible water vapour or ice formation within the shielded room should be treated as indicating a potential leak of gas until such time as the cause of the freezing has been investigated and determined to be safe.

Apart from the risk of a helium leak, the only other major risk presented by the MEG system is the potential for injury to the participant's head or neck while positioning their head within the helmet. If positioning is performed carelessly then the participant's head may strike the inside of the helmet, or their neck may be compressed or rotated with sufficient force to cause injury. While the consequences of such incidents are generally less severe than a helium leak, they have a greater likelihood of occurring and therefore MEG users should always proceed with care when moving the subject's head into or out of the helmet.

Apart from the risks presented by the MEG system itself, there may be additional risks presented by other hardware used in the process of data acquisition. Electrical equipment brought into contact with the participant can present a risk of electrocution if faulty or used incorrectly. Stimulation devices also have the potential to cause harm – for instance, by exposing participants to dangerously high sound volumes or harmful visual stimulation. Any equipment used during MEG recording should therefore be well maintained and only used according to the manufacturer's instructions (and always with the safety and comfort of the participant foremost in mind).

A final issue to be considered when acquiring MEG data is the need for participant monitoring and communication. As the walls of the shielded room generally do not allow direct communication with the participant, there will usually be an intercom system allowing two-way communication with the shielded room and a closed-circuit video system so that the participant can be visually monitored. The participant should be regularly checked on both visually and (where it does not interfere with ongoing data acquisition) verbally. The participant may also be given an alarm that they can press to signal difficulty or distress to the operator.

2.1.3 Magnetic interference

The magnetic field measured by the MEG sensors is not solely generated by the brain. Instead, there are many other sources of magnetism that can contribute to the magnetic field measurements made by MEG. These originate both from the surrounding environment and from physiological processes occurring within parts of the subject's body other than the brain (for instance, due to electrical activity in the heart or muscles). Many of these sources of interference produce magnetic fields that are much stronger (in some cases by several orders of magnitude) than the magnetic field produced by the brain. In data acquired by MEG these sources of interference will introduce data *artefacts*: signals present in the data that do not originate from the brain. It is therefore necessary to minimise these sources of interference in order to minimise their effect on the data.

SQUID sensors are able to measure signals over a wide range of magnetic fields and with SQUID-based systems the objective of magnetic shielding is not to completely eliminate the background magnetic field, but simply to reduce the presence of time-varying magnetic fields that may be difficult to differentiate from the brains own magnetic fields. On the other hand, OPM sensors are maximally sensitive when there is no background magnetic field. Therefore, when acquiring data with OPM sensors, strong levels of both active and passive shielding will generally be required to minimise the background field and maximise the sensitivity of the sensors.

While the magnetic shielding may reduce the impact of magnetic interference originating outside of the shielded room, it cannot reduce magnetic interference from within the room itself. The sources of magnetic interference that might be found inside fall into three broad categories: electrical devices, ferromagnetic materials and physiological processes.

Electrical devices

As we have seen in Chapter 1, all electric currents generate magnetic fields, and therefore all electrical devices have the potential to interfere with MEG measurements. To prevent this, electrical devices are only placed inside the shielded room where unavoidable and when placed in the shielded room they should be kept as far from the MEG sensors as is practically possible. Where possible, non-electrical devices for the transmission of sensory stimulation or behavioural responses should be used. Where an electrical device must be used, direct current (DC) powered devices should be favoured over alternating current (AC) devices to avoid introducing interference at the mains frequency. Particular attention should be paid to the grounding arrangements of any electrical equipment, as the existence of different ground points within a circuit can create ground current loops that can be difficult to locate.

Devices that emit radio-frequency signals (e.g. mobile phones, Wi-Fi-enabled devices) may also act as sources of electromagnetic interference and should generally not be taken into the shielded room. Some electronic devices not intended for the transmission of radio-frequency signals may still nonetheless generate radio-frequency interference if their circuits lack adequate shielding. Electric cables that pass through the waveguides can act as antenna that transmit radio-frequency signals into the shielded room. Attaching a low-pass filter to each cable can limit this problem.

If there is any doubt as to whether or not a particular device may be the source of interference, the simplest test is to observe the MEG data both with and without the device in use and observe if there are any changes to the measured data (viewing the power spectrum of the data can often be particularly informative in this respect).

Ferromagnetism

Some materials become magnetised after exposure to an external magnetic field and retain a magnetic field of their own. This phenomenon is known as *ferromagnetism*. Due to exposure to the Earth's magnetic field and to other sources of magnetism within the environment, all ferromagnetic objects brought into the laboratory environment will carry some residual magnetic field and can potentially produce interference if they are moved within proximity of the MEG sensors (the degree of proximity required to produce detectable interference will depend on the strength of the object's magnetic field).

Ferromagnetic materials can be identified by the fact that they are attracted to magnets. Most materials that contain iron are ferromagnetic (including most forms of stainless steel), whereas materials such as wood, plastic, aluminium, brass and most precious metals are non-ferromagnetic. Unfortunately, many items that are commonly found on participants, such as metal zips, fastenings, buckles, jewellery, bra underwires and the frames of eyeglasses are often ferromagnetic and likely to cause interference. Participants should be asked to remove any suspected ferromagnetic items before entering the shielded room. Metal-free clothing is usually provided for participants to wear to avoid the risk of artefacts from the participant's clothing. Eye make-up may contain ferromagnetic pigments, and therefore will often need to be removed prior to data acquisition. Some items, such as fixed dental work or internally implanted devices, may be ferromagnetic but cannot be easily removed. It may not be possible to record good quality data from participants who have these items on their person.

Ferromagnetic materials will show a greater level of magnetisation (and hence generate more interference) after exposure to an elevated magnetic field, such as in an MRI scanner. Where a MEG recording is performed in conjunction with an MRI scan, it is recommended that MEG should be performed first where possible. It is also recommended to avoid taking items that have been near an MRI scanner into the MEG shielded room.

SQUID sensors are particularly vulnerable to exposure to strong static magnetic fields due to a phenomenon known as *trapped flux*. This is where part of an external magnetic field becomes trapped within the superconducting loop of the SQUID and persists even after the source of field has been removed, impairing the performance of the sensors. To function normally again, the SQUIDs may need to be temporarily warmed above their critical temperature to expel the trapped field. Thus, when working with

SQUID-based MEG system it is generally inadvisable to bring ferromagnetic objects into the shielded room even when data isn't being acquired.

Physiological processes

The brain is not the only source of magnetism in the body, and other physiological magnetic fields can be detected by the MEG sensors and lead to data artefacts. Flexion and extension of muscles involves the flow of electric current within the muscle tissue and where the muscles are close to the MEG sensors (i.e. those in the head and neck) the resulting magnetic fields can produce strong artefacts in the MEG data (Figure 2.2 A). The heartbeat

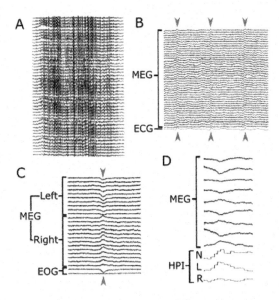

Figure 2.2 Examples of physiological artefacts: (A) Contraction of facial muscles; (B) Cardiac rhythm (ECG also shown for comparison); (C) Eye blink (horizontal and vertical EOG also shown for comparison); (D) Head movements (displacements of head localisation coils are also shown).

produces a distinctive electrical waveform that can be detected by the MEG sensors (indicated by the grey arrows in Figure 2.2 B), particularly by the sensors at the front of the helmet. Eye movements and blinks also produce artefacts (indicated by the grey arrows in Figure 2.2 C) in frontal sensors: as well as the effects of the extraocular muscles, there is a difference in electrical potential between the front and back of the eyeball which leads to a magnetic field being generated when the eye moves. Eye movement and blink artefacts can be increased by the presence of eye make-up containing ferromagnetic pigments, especially if the participant has recently been exposed to a strong magnetic field. Movement of the head and/or torso of the participant will also lead to data artefacts due to movement of the various physiological magnetic fields (including the brain's magnetic field) relative to the sensors (Figure 2.2 D shows a head movement artefact alongside displacement measurements for head localisation coils positioned at the nasion and left and right pre-auricular points).

Because these artefacts are linked to the physiology of the subject, they can never be fully eliminated, but some steps can be taken to reduce them. Instructing the participant to refrain from tensing face and neck muscles and from moving their head can often be effective in reducing artefacts related to muscle and head movements. The use of a visual fixation stimulus can discourage large eye movements and thus reduce eye movement artefacts. Although participants will not be able to prevent themselves from blinking for the entirety of data acquisition (unless the duration is extremely short), instructions to avoid blinking during critical periods of time (for instance during an experimental trial) can sometimes be successful, especially if these are interspersed with other periods (such as between trials or blocks) in which blinking is freely allowed. Where participants are required to make responses during the recording, response methods that might lead the participant to move their head or torso (for instance vocal responses, or motor responses that lead to body movement) should be avoided or, if necessary, delayed so that artefacts occur after measurement of brain responses of interest. Electrophysiological measurements can also be used to monitor, and later remove, artefacts (see Section 3.1.2).

When working with SQUID sensors, a particularly problematic source of artefacts is the movement of the head relative to the sensors: this not only produces transitory artefacts due to the motion itself (as seen in Figure 2.2 D) but can lead to the head changing position relative to the sensors, changing the spatial projection of the brain's magnetic field onto the MEG sensor array. This is generally difficult to correct for, and so head movements should be limited as much as possible during data acquisition. Many participants can remain voluntarily still (to within a few millimetres) for shorter recordings. For longer recordings, or for groups who may find it difficult to remain still (such as young children or individuals suffering from certain medical conditions), it may be necessary to use padding (or other methods) to hold the participant's head as rigidly within the helmet. Head movements can be monitored during data acquisition using the head localisation coils, and verbal feedback may be given to the subject about how well they are keeping their head still.

When working with OPM-MEG the sensors are fixed relative to the scalp, so head movements don't change the position between the sensors and the head. However, head movements move the position of the sensors within the shielded room which can produce artefacts due to inhomogeneities in the background magnetic field. Therefore, subjects should still be encouraged to avoid head movements where possible.

2.1.4 Workflow of data acquisition

To conclude this section, we now present a step-by-step workflow for a typical data acquisition.

1)   *Removal of magnetic items*

The first step is to identify and remove any items from the participant's person that might be ferromagnetic. Ideally participants should be instructed to wear metal-free clothing, or such clothing should be provided for them to change into. They should remove any items containing metal such as jewellery, watches, hair ties, glasses, etc.

2) *Head localisation coils*

To allow accurate measurement of the head's position within the MEG helmet, head localisation coils should be attached to the participant's head. As the head position can vary in three dimensions, a minimum of three coils must be used (additional coils may be attached in order to allow for redundancy).

The coils should be attached to locations on the head which remain fixed regardless of movement (for instance, locations on the jaw or facial muscles are unsuitable). For consistency across participants, it is common for the coils to be placed on anatomical landmarks (or at predetermined locations relative to landmarks). Examples include, the nasion (the small depression above the bridge of the nose), the left and right pre-auricular points (the points in front of the ears where the cheek bone terminates) and the inion (the small protuberance at the base of the skull). The use of anatomical landmarks can also aid in the identification of the location of the coils on the participant's MRI if source localisation is to be performed.

To attach the coils to the skin, medical tape or adhesive rings designed for use with electrodes (or a combination of both) can be used. It is important that the coils are securely attached, so that their position on the head remains fixed throughout the recording.

3) *Electrodes*

Where EEG, EOG, ECG or other electrophysiological measurements are being made alongside MEG, then the electrodes should be attached to the participant. The skin should be cleaned at the sites of electrode placement to remove oils, dead skin and other residue that prevent good electrical contact. Gels containing a mild abrasive are available specifically for this purpose. Some form of conductive gel or paste should generally also be applied between electrode and skin to create a good electrical contact.

4) *Head digitisation*

If MEG data will be coregistered with MRI data (or other imaging data) – for instance, as part of the process of source estimation (see

Chapter 4) – then it is necessary to record the position of the local-isation coils on the head. This is achieved by performing a 3D digit-isation of the participant's scalp surface and of the position of the coils on the scalp. This has conventionally been performed using a stylus connected to a digitiser to measure the spatial coordinates of points across the scalp and of the coils relative to the scalp. More recently, methods based on scanning the head surface using camera-based systems have started to become available. If OPM sensors are used and/or EEG data is to be collected, then the location of each OPM sensor and/or electrode is also recorded as part of this process.

5)   *Positioning the participant*

Next, participants are carefully positioned with their head inside the MEG helmet. Depending on the configuration of the MEG system used, participants may be positioned in seated or supine position. Regardless of the position used, the head must be as close as possible to the sensors to maximise the strength of the measured signal. The participant should be encouraged to make themselves as comfort-able as possible: an uncomfortable position is not only distracting for the participant but could also lead them to move their head or tense their neck muscles, causing data artefacts.

Once the participant is comfortable and in position then the head localisation coils and electrodes can be connected to the MEG system. Any stimulation or response devices should be set up and tested as needed for the recording. The door to the shielded room must then be fully closed, and any equipment for participant monitoring and communication (e.g. alarm system, intercom) should be tested to ensure that it is working correctly.

6)   *Artefact check*

The acquisition software should now be launched to check for the presence of artefacts. The sensor time series will be displayed in real time, and the MEG operator should monitor the display for signs of artefacts. If sources of artefacts have been eliminated from the labora-tory environment and all equipment has undergone prior testing for magnetic interference, remaining artefacts are most likely to originate from the participant themselves.

Some artefacts may only become apparent when the participant makes specific movements, so it can be useful at this stage to instruct them to perform those movements to check that no artefacts appear. Asking them to take a series of deep breaths will help to identify the presence of magnetic material that moves when the participant is breathing, as this will cause the magnetic field to vary in time with each breath. Instructing the participants to repeatedly blink will reveal blink-related artefacts. While all blinks will cause small, transient deflections in the data time series of fronto-temporal sensors (as shown in Figure 2.2 C), the presence of ferromagnetic eye make-up will cause these blink artefacts to be larger than usual. If metallic dental work is present, then asking the participant to slowly open and close their mouth (while trying to otherwise keep their head still) and observing if there are any noticeable changes in the magnetic field can be used to test whether the dental work is ferromagnetic.

While physiological artefacts (such as eye blinks and the cardiac rhythm) typically follow a stereotypical pattern (in terms of their time course and spatial distribution across sensors), other artefacts can often be difficult to identify. The temporal characteristics of the artefact, its distribution across the sensors, and observations of how the participant is moving when the artefact occurs can all provide clues as to the source of the artefact. If the source of the artefact is an item of clothing, then it may be necessary for the participant to be disconnected from the MEG system and leave the shielded room to remove the clothing. This can be awkward and time-consuming, which is why it is always preferable to identify and remove such items beforehand.

7) *Check electrophysiological measures*

If any electrophysiological measures are being collected then the quality of these measurements should also be checked at this time (for EEG it may be preferable to perform any checks before the participant is positioned in the helmet, so that the operator still has access to the scalp in order to make any necessary adjustments). To check for the presence of a faulty electrode or poor electrical contact between the electrode and skin, data time series should be visually inspected for excessive noise levels or the presence of slow drifts in the voltage, and electrode impedance should be measured. Where an electrode has high impedance and/or a noisy time series this suggests a poor electrical contact with the skin surface, the electrode may need to be adjusted to make better physical contact with the skin and/or have further conductive gel/paste applied.

Where electrophysiological recordings are to be used for arte-fact rejection then, if possible, it should be checked visually that the corresponding artefact can be seen clearly in the corresponding traces (for instance, by checking that the heartbeat is visible on the ECG or that the EOG shows a visible deflection when the participant blinks).

8) *Head localisation*

The final step before data acquisition should be to localise the head. Immediately prior to head localisation, participants should be verbally and/or visually (i.e. using instructions on the screen) reminded that from this point onwards they should keep their heads as still as possible until instructed otherwise. The head localisation coils are then activated from the data acquisition computer so that their position within the helmet can be measured. If excessive head movement is observed at this point, then the participant may need a further reminder to remain still.

9) *Data acquisition*

Once head localisation has been completed, data acquisition should commence as soon as possible to minimise the time that the participant is required to remain still. Visually, the data acquisition software may not look different during acquisition: the data time series still appear on the display but whereas before they were shown purely for visualisation purposes, they will now be saved to file. If the participant is undergoing an experimental task, then the task should be started.

It is advisable to monitor the sensor time series during acquisition to watch for the presence of any unexpected artefacts. It should also be checked that event triggers are being acquired by the MEG acquisition software. If the triggers are not collected – or are collected incorrectly – then it may not be possible to accurately determine the timing of experimental events within the data, which will make it impossible to perform subsequent data analysis. If a closed-circuit video system is present then this should be regularly monitored, both for safety reasons and to ensure that the participant is remaining alert and is continuing to perform experimental tasks as instructed. If head position is being acquired continuously then the operator will be also able to monitor head motion in real time, and this should be regularly checked to ensure that the participant is staying sufficiently still.

10) *End of session*

Once all the planned acquisition protocols have been completed then the acquisition session comes to an end. Localisation coils and electrodes can be disconnected from the MEG system and the subject brought out of the shielded room. To maintain good hygiene, some labs may require that any parts of the MEG system that have been in direct contact with the participants skin are cleaned with disinfecting wipes. Electrodes should be cleaned as per the manufacturer's instructions.

2.2 Experimental design

The constraints on the design of experimental protocols for MEG are somewhat different from those of other types of behavioural experiment, and therefore it is often inadvisable (and sometimes not possible) to simply transfer a task, unaltered, from another setting. MEG experiments generally need to conform to one of two experimental designs: event-related or block-based. In this section we will look at the principles behind each of these designs, while exploring the critical role event triggers play in recording information about the timing of experimental events.

2.2.1 Event-related experimental designs

Many of the brain signals that can be measured using MEG are reflected in a series of short duration responses occurring at a fixed latency relative to task-related events such as the onset or offset of sensory stimuli or behavioural responses. Measurement of these responses are often best made using what is known as an *event-related* experimental design. In this design, the experiment is structured around a series of trials containing one or more events that elicit task-related brain responses. Figure 2.3 illustrates a series of two trials from an event-related experiment where each trial contains three time periods: a fixation period (to be used as a baseline; see below), the presentation of a stimulus (here represented by two conditions corresponding to two different facial emotions) and a response period (where the subject is required to make a behavioural response to each stimulus).

In event-related designs, the occurrence of each event is signalled to the MEG system by an event trigger (see Section 2.2.3), allowing data to be analysed relative to the timing of each event. Brain responses that occur at a consistent time relative to the event (and therefore can be said to be time-locked to the event) will occur at the same latency relative to the corresponding trigger and can therefore be measured by analysing the data relative to the time of the trigger.

Event-related designs naturally lend themselves to the measurement of brain signals related to sensory or motor processes that have a consistent relationship in time to a particular form of sensory stimulation or behavioural response. It is also possible to measure

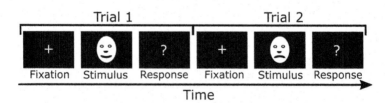

Figure 2.3 Illustration of trials from an event-related experiment.

signals related to cognitive processes, provided that they are time-locked to an experimental event. Behavioural experiments designed to measure reaction times particularly lend themselves to event-related designs, as the requirement to respond rapidly will tend to impose a degree of consistency in the timing of the corresponding event-related brain responses. On the other hand, brain signals which are variable in their timing to experimental events usually cannot be measured using event-related designs.

The timing and duration of events within a trial will influence which event-related responses can be measured. For instance, briefly presented stimuli are likely to be processed with less depth than stimuli presented for a longer duration, and therefore may be less likely to evoke high-level sensory and cognitive processes and their associated responses. This will also interact with the experimental task: simple sensory stimuli may only elicit basic sensory responses and therefore may require only a brief presentation, whereas stimuli that engage higher-level sensory and cognitive processing may produce a longer series of responses when presented for a longer duration. Event-related responses are triggered not only by the onset of stimuli but by their offset as well. Thus, the time interval between stimuli must be long enough to prevent responses to the offset of each stimulus overlapping in time with responses to the onset of the subsequent stimulus. Most analyses of event-related responses require measurement of the response relative to a baseline period during which no event-related responses occur, and so a baseline time interval must also be factored into the trial structure.

The timing of any behavioural responses also needs to be planned with care. Button presses and other motor responses will generate their own event-related responses, not only at the time of the behavioural response itself but also beforehand due to preparatory processes. If these signals overlap with event-related responses to stimuli, the two types of response may be difficult to separate. One possible solution to this problem is to use experiments that do not require any behavioural response, but this comes with the disadvantage that it is more difficult to determine if the participant has remained alert and engaged with the experience. Other possible solutions are to require the subject to delay their response to an inter-trial interval, to require responses only in a small proportion of trials that can then be discarded prior to data analysis, or to require a response after all trials are completed (for instance, by asking participants to count certain events and report their number at the end of the task). Where it is not possible to separate stimulus presentation and behavioural responses in time (for instance, if the task requires the measurement of reaction times) then it is recommended to counter-balance responses across stimuli to avoid the introduction of response confounds.

Measurement of event-related brain responses usually requires averaging the MEG data across multiple trials. In general, the more trials included in the average, the more accurate the measurements of the corresponding response will be. However, when deciding on the number of trials, the total duration of the experiment must also be taken into consideration. The duration of the experiment becomes longer as the number of trials increases, and participants will increasingly struggle to maintain attention to the experimental task and to limit head movements. For longer event-related experiments it may therefore be beneficial to break the trials into short blocks separated with short breaks.

2.2.2 Block experimental designs

While event-related designs are best suited to the measurement of task-related responses of short duration, other brain responses may be sustained continuously in response to a continuous experimental task (for instance to continuous sensory stimulation or continuous performance of a cognitive or behavioural task). These responses may be better measured using a block design (sometimes also known as a boxcar design), where the subject performs a continuous task across an extended block of time. Each experimental condition can then be performed repeatedly across multiple blocks, inter-leaved across conditions. Figure 2.4 shows an example of the structure of block design containing blocks of three conditions: visual stimulation, auditory stimulation and a rest condition in which there is no stimulation.

In block designs, event triggers are used to signal the onset of each block, so that data can be averaged across blocks. As with

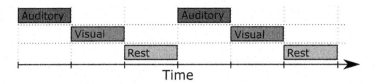

Figure 2.4 Illustration of a block experimental design.

event-related designs, measurement of brain responses in block designs is often based on comparison with a baseline time period during which no task-related responses are present. In block designs, this can be achieved by including some blocks containing no task (such as the rest blocks in Figure 2.4) that can be contrasted with task blocks, or by including an inter-block interval at the start of each block that can then be used as a baseline for the corresponding block. Because block designs involve fewer intervals in which the task is not performed, they are therefore often shorter in duration than the equivalent event-related design.

Block designs are generally less sensitive than event-related designs to variations of the timing of the response across repetitions. As long as a particular brain response varies between blocks it can be detected by contrasting between blocks, even if the precise timing of the response varies between blocks. However, collapsing data across time within a block removes information about the timing of brain responses, and thus measurements of response timing generally must be performed using event-related designs.

Some short duration brain signals in response to sensory stimuli or behavioural responses that might usually be measured in event-related designs can often also be measured in block designs by repetition of the stimulus or response within a block. The event-related response can then be measured as a sustained response at the frequency of repetition (or at integer multiples of that frequency). For example, presenting a sensory stimulus four times a second should generate four event-related responses a second which would be equivalent to a 4 Hz continuous response. This is often known as the *steady-state evoked response*. In a related technique – known as *frequency tagging* – different stimuli (or parts of a single stimulus) are modulated at different frequencies, and the brain responses to each stimulus can separated be measuring the signal at each corresponding frequency.

2.2.3 Event triggers

The timing of events and blocks are not directly observable within the MEG data itself (except in rare cases where the timing of an event corresponds to a particular electrophysiological response recorded with the data) but are instead signalled by digital (or, more rarely, analog) triggers that coincide with them. Thus, the design of event triggers is of critical importance for subsequent analysis of the data.

Event triggers are signals generated either directly by the peripheral devices involved in stimulus presentation or response measurement, or indirectly by the stimulus computer, and transmitted to the MEG acquisition electronics in order to be recorded with the MEG data. Most commonly, triggers are transmitted digitally using a system known as *transistor-transistor logic* (*TTL*) which allows the transmission of different integer values. The trigger channel is set to zero when no information is transmitted and takes on non-zero values when a trigger is sent, where each different value represents a different trigger type. These trigger values are usually transmitted as short duration pulses, so that the timing of the pulse can represent the timing of the corresponding event. Less commonly, triggers can be transmitted by assigning values to certain states of an analog input signal from a peripheral device or based on a physiological measure.

Figure 2.5 illustrates digital triggers for a hypothetical task in which participants respond to one of two stimulus types (vertical or horizontal images) by pressing one of two response buttons. The trigger value (represented by the y-axis) is set to zero except at times when an event occurs. In this example, the onsets of the vertical and horizontal stimuli correspond to trigger values of 1 and 2 respectively, and the onsets of the two response buttons are represented by trigger values of 3 and 4. Data can then be analysed with respect to these triggers in order to measure event-related responses time-locked to the trigger (or in block designs, the triggers can be used to indicate the onset of each block).

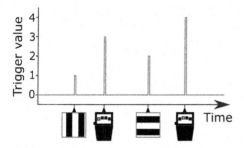

Figure 2.5 Illustration of event triggers.

The different trigger values can be used to signal different types of event (e.g. stimulus onsets or behavioural responses) but also variations within one event type (e.g. different stimulus conditions or response options). In the example study shown in Figure 2.5, this would make it possible to analyse separate event-related responses to the two stimulus conditions (or the two response options) as different trigger values are used to represent the two stimulus conditions. Therefore, when designing a new experiment, it is important to ensure that every type of event (or block) that may later be analysed has a unique trigger value assigned to it. If an event does not have a corresponding trigger, it will generally be impossible to later analyse the data relative to that event.

Although ideally the trigger should be recorded in the data at the exact time of the stimulus/response event, in practice there are almost always timing differences between the trigger and the event itself. While electrical transmission can be considered instantaneous, any interactions with electronic components (including hardware components of the stimulus computer) potentially introduce delays to either stimulus presentation, the measurement of behavioural responses or to the transmission of the corresponding event triggers. The software used for running the experimental paradigm may also introduce delays, either due to the intrinsic limitations of the software or due to user errors in implementing the experiment. Other software processes running on the stimulus computer (including processes related to the operating system) can also introduce timing delays if they compete for computing resources with the experimental software. Delays can also be occurred by the physical transmission of stimuli. The most common example of this is where auditory stimuli are transmitted via pneumatic tubes to the participant. Sound requires 3 ms to travel along each metre of tubing and so, depending on the length of the tubing used, a proportional delay will be introduced between the physical generation of a sound and the sound reaching the ear.

In some cases, the difference in timing between an experimental event and the physical presentation of a stimulus can be measured (for instance using a photodiode to measure the onset of visual stimulus, or a sound meter to measure the onset of a sound). Where these differences are consistent across presentations, the delay can be corrected for by shifting the data forwards or backwards in time by a fixed interval. A more serious problem occurs if the timing difference varies across presentations, as this will introduce uncertainty to the timing of events within the data. Therefore, whenever possible, hardware and software designed for reliable event timing should be used for conducting experiments with MEG.

2.2.4 Summary

MEG is frequently used as a method to measure brain activity while subjects perform one or more experimental tasks. In this section we have seen that experiments with MEG data acquisition usually follow either an event-related or block design. Event-related designs involve subjects performing a series of experimental trials and are therefore best used to measure short duration responses that are time-locked to experimental events occurring within the trials. Conversely, blocks designs involve subjects undergoing as series of blocks containing continuous (or periodically repeated) stimulation or a continuous task and are best suited to measure task-related responses that are extended over the length of a block.

For both types of experimental design, analysis of the data must be performed relative to specific events occurring within the experiment: either the timing of events within a trial in event-related designs or the timing of blocks in block designs. The timing of these events is transmitted to the MEG system using event triggers. Ensuring that these event triggers contain the information necessary to subsequently identify the type and timing of these events is necessary for successful analysis of task-related brain responses.

Further reading

Gross, J. et al. (2013). Good practice for conducting and reporting MEG research, *NeuroImage, 65*, 349–363. https://doi.org/10.1016/j.neuroim age.2012.10.001

Mosher, J. C., & Funke, M. E. (2020). Towards best practices in clinical magnetoencephalography: patient preparation and data acquisition, *Journal of Clinical Neurophysiology, 37*(6), 498–507. https://doi.org/10.1097/WNP.0000000000000542

Parkkonen, L., & Salmelin, R. (2010). Measurements. In P. C. Hansen, M. L. Kringelbach, & R. Salmelin (Eds.), *MEG: An introduction to methods*, 65–74. Oxford University Press. https://doi.org/10.1093/acprof:oso/9780195307238.003.0003

Puce A., & Hämäläinen, M. S. (2017) A review of issues related to data acquisition and analysis in EEG/MEG studies. *Brain Sciences, 7*(6), 58. https://doi.org/10.3390/brainsci7060058

Salmelin, R., & Parkkonen, L., (2010). Experimental design. In P. C. Hansen, M. L. Kringelbach, & R. Salmelin (Eds.), *MEG: An introduction to methods*, 75–82. Oxford University Press. https://doi.org/10.1093/acprof:oso/9780195307238.003.0004

Stephen, J. M. (2014). Designing MEG experiments. In S. Supek & C. J. Aine (Eds.), *Magnetoencephalography: From signals to dynamic cortical networks*, 41–71. Springer. https://doi.org/10.1007/978-3-642-33045-2_5

Part II

Analysing the data

Chapter 3

Analysing data time series

Having looked in Part I at what MEG measures, and how it is measured, in Part II of the book we will look at how MEG data can be analysed in order to provide information about the various brain processes that give rise to the brain's magnetic field.

While acquisition of MEG data is usually a fairly simple process, analysis of the data is a much more complex matter. There are a wide variety of methods used for analysis of MEG data, with new techniques being added frequently. As MEG is acquired as a series of measurements over time, in its native format the data can be analysed with respect to time in what is known as the *time domain*. However, the data can be transformed into the *frequency domain*, where data is represented as a series of measurements varying with respect to frequency, or into the *time–frequency domain*, where the data is represented as varying with respect to both time and frequency. Different aspects of temporal information present in the data can be explored, and different analyses of the data can be performed, in each of these three different domains.

The possibilities for analysis increase even further when we consider the spatial information present in the data. MEG data is collected across an array of sensors positioned outside the head, and the data can be analysed with respect to the spatial distribution of the magnetic field over these sensors, in what is known as *sensor space*. However, there are also a variety of techniques that allow estimation of the spatial distribution of the source currents in the brain that gave rise to the measurements of the magnetic field made by the sensors.

DOI: 10.4324/9781315205175-5

Data can then be analysed with respect to the spatial distribution of these currents, in what is known as *source space*.

Thus, the reason that there are a large range of methods for analysing MEG data is that there are potentially six different combinations of the three temporal domains and two spaces that the MEG data can be represented in. The range of measures that can be extracted from MEG data is therefore larger and more complex than for most other techniques. As a result, it can often be difficult to decide which are the most appropriate methods for analysing a particular data set, especially for those starting out with MEG. One of the aims of this part of the book is to help the reader better understand which methods are best suited to which situations.

To begin the process, in Section 3.1 of this chapter we will look at some of the data preprocessing steps that can be used to format and clean the data prior to data analysis. We will then look at how MEG data time series from individual sensors (or sources when working in source space) can be analysed, first in the time domain (Section 3.2) and then in the frequency and time–frequency domains (Section 3.3).

3.1 Data preprocessing

After data has been collected, it is typically necessary to apply one or more processing steps to format and clean the raw data ahead of analysis. These steps are known collectively as data *preprocessing*. In this section we will give an overview of three of the most commonly used preprocessing steps.

3.1.1 Epoching

As mentioned in the previous chapter, analysis of MEG data normally takes place with respect to an experimental event. When this is the case, the raw data is split into a series of shorter segments around each occurrence of that event. Each of these segments is known as an *epoch*, and the process of segmenting the data into epochs is often known as *epoching* the data. In experimental studies, an epoch generally corresponds to a trial (in event-related designs) or a block (in block designs) but can correspond to other periods of time (for instance, where an event is repeated multiple times in a trial, each trial may be segmented into multiple epochs corresponding to each occurrence of the event). Figure 3.1 shows an illustration of a continuous data set (upper panel) segmented into three epochs (lower panels) based on three event triggers (trigger times shown by the dashed grey lines).

To facilitate averaging of data across epochs, each epoch is of a fixed length, with the experimental event used to define the epoch occurring at the same time sample within each epoch. The precise start and end time of the epochs relative to the event are chosen to include time periods containing event-related responses of interest, and any required baseline time interval. In the example shown in Figure 3.1 each epoch is defined as starting one second before the event of interest and ending one and a half seconds following the

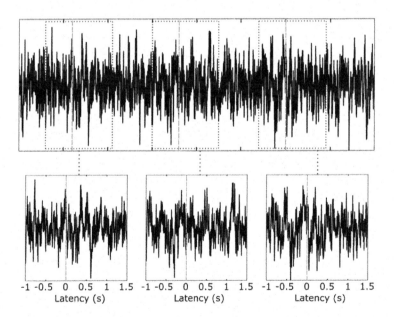

Figure 3.1 Illustration of epoching. The lower panels show epochs segmented from the continuous data series shown in the upper panel.

event. The timing of data samples (and the brain responses contained within those samples) within each epoch are typically characterised by their *latency* relative to the experimental event. Thus, in the example shown in Figure 3.1 the first and last samples of each epoch would correspond to latencies of -1 s and 1.5 s respectively.

3.1.2 Artefact removal

As explored in the previous chapter, there are many sources of magnetic interference that introduce artefacts to the data. While ideally these are minimised at the time of data acquisition, it is never possible to eliminate all artefacts from the data (especially those which are physiological in origin, such as eye blink and cardiac artefacts). It may be possible to ignore these remaining artefacts if they don't interfere with brain signals of interest (for instance, eye blink artefacts mainly effect frontal sensors, and hence may have a limited impact on analyses involving posterior sensors). However, in other circumstances it may be necessary to remove (or at least attenuate) some of the remaining artefacts from the data during preprocessing.

Where data is formatted into epochs, a crude approach to removing artefacts is simply to reject any epoch that contains a data artefact. This can be achieved either by manually inspecting the data to visually identify artefacts, or by applying automated procedures that flag epochs as containing an artefact if some quantitative measure is exceeded (such as whether the maximum or minimum of the epoch exceeds some threshold). This can be an effective approach for artefacts that occur infrequently and are restricted to a small number of epochs (such as muscle or head motion artefacts). The drawback of this method is that it reduces the number of epochs available for subsequent analysis and, for frequently occurring artefacts (such as cardiac and blink artefacts), can lead to most (or even all) epochs being excluded from the data. This method also cannot be applied if the analysis is performed on continuous (i.e. non-epoched) data.

A more sophisticated approach is to use methods that attempt to remove artefacts from the data while leaving the data otherwise unchanged. There are several approaches to achieving this, each with different strengths and weaknesses.

If an independent measure of an artefact is available (for instance measurements of eye movements and blinks from EOG or of the cardiac rhythm from ECG) then it is possible to use linear regression methods to identify the contribution of the artefact to the data time series and to regress the artefacts out of the data (Gratton et al., 1983). The downside of this approach is that brain signals may also be accidentally removed from the data if they are correlated with the measure used for regression.

Where no independent measure of the artefact is available (or the measure is suspected to be correlated with brain signals), an alternative approach is the class of methods known as *blind source separation*. These techniques attempt to separate the data time series into different components (where each component has a fixed distribution across the sensors) based purely on the statistical properties of the data. The most frequently used of these techniques is *independent component analysis* (ICA) which, as the name suggests, separates data into a set of statistically independent time series (Ikeda & Toyama, 2000). Assuming that the time course of brain signals and artefacts are statistically independent from each other, these should be separated into different components, and it should be possible to remove artefacts from the data simply identifying and subtracting the corresponding components.

The strength of blind source separation techniques is that they do not require any information about the artefacts present in the data (hence why the techniques are described as 'blind') and so in theory can be used to remove any kind of artefact. However, a drawback is that it is generally necessary for the user to identify the components that contain artefacts, meaning that it can generally only be applied to artefacts that are visually identifiable. There is also no guarantee that brain signals and artefacts will be perfectly separated into different components, and this means that, as with linear regression, brain signal may inadvertently be removed along with the artefact.

A final set of approaches are the signal space methods. These approaches assume that artefacts and brain signals have a different spatial distribution across the sensor array. If the spatial distribution of artefacts can be identified, then signals present in the data that follow that distribution can be removed from the data while leaving other signals unaffected. There are two commonly used methods for achieving this.

In the first case, the spatial distribution of the artefacts can be estimated from a data set which contains only the artefacts to be removed (for instance, an 'empty-room' recording where there was no participant present), and signals with this distribution can then be removed from the data (Uusitalo & Ilmoniemi, 1997). This is known as *signal-space projection* (SSP). The strength of this technique is that, like blind source separation, it is entirely data driven and requires no additional information. However, the weakness is that it can only remove artefacts that can be measured separately from brain signals (such as environmental noise). As with blind source separation there is also a risk that brain signals may be removed from the data if their spatial distribution across the sensors is not fully separable from the spatial distribution of the artefacts to be removed.

The second method uses the known physical properties of magnetic fields to calculate the spatial distributions of fields originating from outside of the helmet, and then removing signals with that distribution (Taulu et al., 2004). This is known as *signal-space separation* (SSS). The advantage of this latter approach is that it can in theory attenuate all artefacts that originate from outside of the helmet. The downside is that the method requires precise information about the geometry of the MEG sensor array, and this information may not always be available.

3.1.3 Temporal filtering

Another commonly used preprocessing step that aids in reducing the contribution of artefacts and other noise signals from the data (such as measurement noise introduced by the MEG hardware and intrinsic noise within the brain signals themselves) is temporal filtering. Time series data can be represented as the sum of a series of periodic components of different frequency (for more detail see the next chapter). Filtering is the process of supressing signals within the data at a specific range of frequencies, while leaving signals at other frequencies unaltered. Because the frequency content of noise signals may sometimes differ from those of brain signals, temporal filtering can be used to selectively reduce noise while leaving brain signals unaffected. In addition, where multiple brain signals are present at different frequencies, filtering can be used to focus on one or more signals of interest by supressing signals at other frequencies.

Temporal filters filter out signals within a frequency range known as the *stopband* while preserving signals at the remaining frequencies, whose range is known as the *passband*. Temporal filters can pass signal above (*high-pass* filtering) or below (*low-pass* filtering) *a cut-off* frequency. Low-pass filtering filters out high frequency components of the data. This increases the smoothness of the data in time (Figure 3.2). Conversely, high-pass filtering filters out low frequency components of the data, reducing slow changes in the data (Figure 3.2). Low- and high-pass filtering can also be performed simultaneously so that signal is passed at frequencies between two frequency cut-offs. This is known as band-pass filtering.

A further class of filter is the *band-stop* filter, which filters out signal between the frequency cut-offs while passing signal outside the cut-offs. There are two types of band-stop filter: the *notch filter* which filters out signal from a single stopband, and a *comb filter* which has multiple stopbands at integer multiples of a specific frequency. In MEG data analysis, band-stop filters are useful

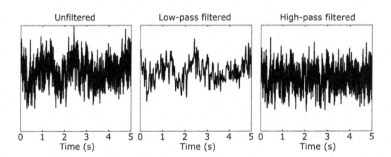

Figure 3.2 The effects of filtering. The left panel shows five seconds of raw unfiltered data. The central and right panels show the same data after low-pass and high-pass filtering respectively.

for removing artefacts that are present at a narrow frequency range, such as the artefact due to the electrical mains signal (also known as the *powerline* signal) which is present at either 50 or 60 Hz (depending on the local mains frequency), as well as at some integer multiples of that frequency.

An ideal filter would completely remove all signal within its stopband while leaving signal within its passband unaffected, but such a filter is not achievable in practice. Instead, filters have a *transition band* around the frequency cut-off in which the filter response has a gradual *roll off* (Figure 3.3). Some filters may also exhibit *ripple*, meaning that their response functions may not be flat in the pass and stop bands (Figure 3.3) and therefore do not pass or attenuate signal evenly at all frequencies within those bands. Different filters have different roll offs and exhibit different amounts of ripple as well as varying in other respects, such as whether they are causal (each time sample is affected only by previous time samples) or acausal (time samples can affected by subsequent as well as previous time samples) and whether they exhibit a finite impulse response (meaning that the time series eventually returns to zero after a brief input) or an infinite impulse response (meaning that the time series may remain non-zero indefinitely after a brief input). Therefore decisions about which filters to use must be taken with care, especially as filtering

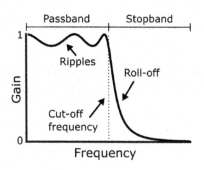

Figure 3.3 Annotated response function of a low-pass filter. The filter gain shows the proportion of signal power passed by the filter at the corresponding frequency.

can distort the data time series in various ways (de Cheveigné & Nelken, 2019).

MEG acquisition hardware will usually allow temporal filters to be applied at the time of data acquisition (this is known as *online filtering*). However, because the filtering process cannot be reversed (due to the permanent loss of information from the data), it is generally recommended that filtering be applied after the data has been acquired (this is known as *offline filtering*) and that a copy of the unfiltered data be retained in case the filtering later needs to be undone. Offline temporal filtering can introduce distortions of the data at edges of the time series, known as *edge artefacts*. For this reason, filtering may sometimes be applied prior to epoching, so that edge artefacts only occur at the start and end of the full data time series, rather than occurring at the start and end of every epoch.

3.1.4 Summary

Data preprocessing consists in a series of processing steps applied to data prior to analysis. This commonly involves splitting the data into a series of short segments known as epochs, where each epoch contains a single instance of an experimental event of interest. Preprocessing also often involves applying one or more methods for removing artefacts from the data and/or the use of temporal filtering to attenuate signals (both artefacts and brain responses) occurring outside of specific frequencies of interest.

3.2 The time domain

Most MEG data analysis involves analysis of time series data. When analysing the data in sensor space this involves analysing the time series of magnetic field measurements made at one or more sensors, while when analysing the data in source space this involves analysing the time series of source currents at one or more locations in the brain. In general, the same set of time series analysis techniques can be applied to the data regardless of whether data is analysed in sensor or source space, and therefore the analysis techniques we describe in this (and the following) section can be applied to both types of data.

Where time series data is analysed in its native format as a series of measurements of data over time, then analysis is said to be performed in the time domain. In this section we will look at the commonly used approaches to analysing MEG data in the time domain.

3.2.1 Data analysis in the time domain

MEG data are acquired as a series of measurements of the magnetic field across time samples, where the *amplitude* of the signal at each sample corresponds to measurements of the field strength at that instant in time (or to measurements of dipole moment when working in source space), usually relative to some baseline (see below). This data can then be used to measure event-related responses: brain responses that are time-locked to an experimental event.

In general, event-related responses tend to be weak relative to sources of noise present in the data (these sources of noise include the various sources of magnetic interference described in Section 2.1.3, measurement noise introduced by the MEG sensors and acquisition hardware, and the inherent noisiness of the brain signals themselves) and therefore usually cannot be measured from individual epochs. Instead, data generally needs to be averaged across epochs to reliably measure event-related responses. If data epochs are aligned to the corresponding event, then the event-related responses should occur at the same latency in each epoch and will average together across epochs. By contrast, the amplitude of noise signals at each sample will be variable across epochs and therefore will tend to cancel out by averaging (the signal-to-noise ratio increasing by a factor of the square root of the number of epochs used to calculate the average). This means that averaging time series across epochs should suppress signals present in the data that are not time-locked (or, in the case of periodic signals, not phase-locked – see Section 3.3.4 and Chapter 5) to the experimental event, while time-locked responses should be unaffected.

In EEG, where this technique of measuring brain signals from event-related averages was first used, the average time series typically contain a series of time-locked increases and decreases of the scalp potential, known as *event-related potentials* (ERPs). In MEG, similar event-related changes in the magnetic field are observed in the average time series and are known as *event-related fields* (ERFs). An example of an event-related field in response to visual presentation of face stimuli is shown in Figure 3.4. Analysis of event-related fields (or the source currents that generate those fields) is the most frequently used approach to the analysis of MEG data in the time domain.

Note, however, that the rationale for measuring event-related responses by averaging across epochs assumes that those responses have a consistent latency within each epoch. This means that variability of the timing of the responses – this can be due to variability in the lag between an event and its corresponding trigger (as described in Section 2.2.3) or due to intrinsic variability of the response itself – can lead to inaccurate results. The presence of variability will tend to smooth the average event-related response, and this in turn will tend to reduce the amplitude of the peaks of the response and may cause partial cancellation of the response where peaks of opposite sign are smoothed together. This is illustrated in Figure 3.4 where plots B and C show the response plotted in A, but with the timing of the event onset varying across epochs by a random interval in the range ±25

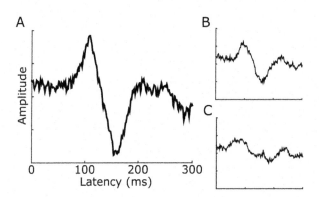

Figure 3.4 (A) Data from a single MEG sensor averaged across a series of trials relative to the onset of a stimulus. (B) & (C) The same average time series when timing of the stimulus onset varies randomly across epochs in the range ±25 ms and ±50 ms respectively.

ms and ±50 ms respectively. Thus, when measuring event-related responses it is important to use experimental designs that generate brain responses that are consistent in their timing across trials, and to ensure that this timing is accurately signalled by the corresponding event triggers.

A second problem encountered when measuring the amplitude of event-related responses is that, because the strength of background magnetic field during acquisition is never zero and because some sources of noise have non-zero mean, MEG time series data usually does not vary around zero, but around some non-zero offset. The amplitude measured at each sample is therefore a combination of both the event-related response and this offset. To accurately measure the amplitude of the event-related response, it is necessary to remove this offset by measuring the mean amplitude of the data within a baseline time interval and subtracting the mean from all samples. This process is known as *baseline correction* and when applied means that the amplitude at each sample is measured as change from the baseline amplitude.

To illustrate why this is necessary, Figure 3.5 A shows an example of average time series of two stimulus conditions in which the amplitude of each condition has a different offset from zero. Comparisons of the event-related responses between the two conditions will be confounded by the fact that measurements of the difference in amplitude between conditions will include differences in this offset as

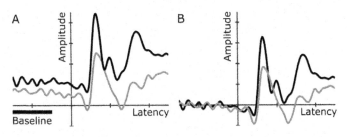

Figure 3.5 Average time series showing the event-related responses to two stimulus conditions, shown before (A) and after (B) baseline correction.

well as difference in the event-related responses. Figure 3.5 B shows the two average time series after the mean amplitude of the baseline time window shown in Figure 3.5 A has been subtracted from each of the time series. After baseline correction the amplitudes of the event-related responses are now measured relative to the same offset and therefore can be directly compared.

It is important that the time interval used as the baseline does not contain any event-related responses so that these do not contribute to the baseline amplitude that is subtracted from each data sample. For stimulus events, event-related responses should always occur after the stimulus onset (unless the stimulus elicits preparatory responses), so it is usually reasonable to assume that time intervals occurring before stimulus onset are free of event-related responses and can be safely used for the baseline. For motor and other behavioural responses, the time interval prior to the event is likely to include preparatory responses, and so the baseline period is generally chosen to be earlier in time to avoid including these responses.

Once the data has been averaged and baseline corrected, statistical analysis can then be applied to the average time series. In theory a separate analysis can be performed for each time sample to detect for the presence of an event-related response (or a difference in responses between conditions) at that sample (this corresponds to a mass univariate analysis of the data, as described in Chapter 4). However, performing statistical tests at each sample requires many statistical comparisons (especially if the statistical testing is also being performed across sensors or sources as well as across time samples), and correcting for multiple comparisons in order to achieve a desired rate of false positives will cause a reduction in the power to detect statistical effects (see Section 4.3 for more details). For this reason, event-related responses are usually not analysed in this way (although see Groppe et al. (2011) for an argument in favour of mass univariate analysis of event-related responses).

The event-related response typically consists in a series of time-limited increases and decreases in the amplitude of the magnetic field, and for analysis purposes these changes in amplitude are often treated as discrete components of the response. Many of these components of the event-related response have been identified in the EEG literature, where a vast body of research has identified and catalogued components of the event-related potential and their links to specific brain processes (Kappenman & Luck, 2012). These potentials are often known by alphanumeric descriptors such as N70 or P3, where the initial letter describes the polarity of the potential (i.e. whether it is a positive or negative potential when measured at the scalp) and the number describes either the approximate timing of the potential (thus, the N70 would usually occur around 70 ms) or the numeric order of the particular event-related potential (thus, the P3 would be the third positive component following the event of interest). Alternatively, the components are sometimes known by descriptive terms, such as 'the mismatch negativity' or 'the vertex positive potential' Many of these responses can also be measured using MEG. Because source currents produce magnetic fields that have both negative and positive components, event-related fields are often labelled by the polarity of the corresponding event-related potential (with the label followed by a lower case or m to indicate that it is a magnetic field component rather than an electrical potential) or the polarity is replaced by the letter M (thus, the MEG equivalent to the P100 potential may be labelled the P100m or the M100).

Rather than analysing MEG average time series separately at each sample, it is therefore common to measure properties of these components instead. For instance, the amplitude of an individual component may be quantified by measuring the peak or average amplitude within a pre-defined time window (and across a pre-defined set of sensors). Statistical comparisons can then be performed on this single measure of amplitude per component, rather than across the multiple time samples that make up that component, leading to fewer statistical comparisons. Alternatively, where the objective is to measure the timing, rather than strength, of an event-related response, the timing of the corresponding component can be measured based on the latency of the peak or (in order to quantify the onset rather than peak of the response) the latency at which the response reaches a certain fraction of the peak amplitude.

In theory, the latency of brain responses can be measured to the precision defined by the sampling interval of the data (e.g. the response timing can be measured to the nearest millisecond if the sampling interval is equal to 1 ms). However, because low-pass filtering (including anti-alias filtering) smooths the data in time (and therefore introduces some degree of dependency between neighbouring samples), the effective time resolution of the data will be determined by the cut-off frequency of any low-pass filters applied during any online or offline filtering. Additionally, although high-pass filtering does not affect the time resolution of the data, it can shift the timing and shape of event-related responses (Acunzo et al., 2012). Thus, when measuring the timing of event-related responses, care must be taken to ensure the results are not affected by any temporal filtering that has been applied to the data.

We will look at some examples of how event-related responses are measured and analysed in the time domain in the next chapter. A more detailed discussion on the quantification and analysis of the components of the event-related response can also be found in Chapter 6 of Luck (2014).

3.2.2 Summary

In this section we have looked at how MEG data can be analysed with respect to changing amplitude (of either the field strength in sensor space or the dipole moment in source space) over time. This is the time domain representation of the data. This approach can be used to measure event-related responses: changes in the magnetic field (or source current) occurring with a consistent latency relative to an experimental event. Analysis of event-related responses in the time domain typically requires the data to be averaged across epochs, in order to average out noise signals which are not time-locked to the experimental event. Event-related responses in the average time series can then be measured and analysed based on their amplitude or latency, depending on the specific hypothesis to be tested.

3.3 The frequency and time–frequency domains

While the time domain forms a core part of MEG analysis (and indeed some researchers may never need to go beyond time domain analysis), there are many signals of interest that are difficult to analyse

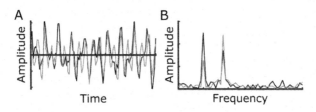

Figure 3.6 Example data from two stimulus conditions represented in the time (A) and frequency (B) domains.

when data is represented as a series of samples with respect to time. We can see an illustration of this in Figure 3.6 A, which shows two time series representing two different experimental conditions. There are clearly differences between the series, but these differences are distributed across time and do not appear to be limited to a particular time interval. Both time series appear to contain repetitive structure, however, meaning that they may be well represented by the combination of a series of periodic components of different frequency. Indeed, if we represent the data as a series of measurements over frequency (Figure 3.6 B) then we can see that the differences in the two conditions can be largely explained by differences in the signals at just two frequencies (we will see how this representation was created in the next section). Thus, we can see that data containing periodic signals may be more clearly understood when analysed as a series of measurements over frequency rather than time, or (as we shall later) over a combination of time and frequency. Data represented in these ways are said to be represented in the frequency domain and time–frequency domain, respectively.

Many brain responses measured by MEG are periodic in nature, either because they reflect repeated event-related responses to repetitive sensory stimulation or behavioural responses, or because the source currents themselves are intrinsically periodic (for examples of the latter, see Chapter 5). These signals are therefore most appropriately analysed in the frequency or time–frequency domains. In this section we will look at how data can be analysed in each of these two domains, starting with the frequency domain.

3.3.1 The Fourier transform

In order to analyse data in the frequency domain, the data must first be transformed from a series of measurements over time into a series of measurements across frequency. This is usually achieved by performing a mathematical transform known as the Fourier transform. This transform works on the basis that any data time series can be represented as the sum of a unique set of sine waves of different frequency (where frequency is the number of cycles of the sine wave per second and is measured in Hz). Figure 3.7 illustrates this by showing some periodic time series and the corresponding sets of sine waves that can be summed to create those time series. The Fourier transform consists of decomposing a data time series into the corresponding sine waves, and representing the data based on the parameters of those waves.

The frequencies that must be used to characterise the chosen time series are those that fit the data with an integer number of cycles. Thus, the lowest frequency sine wave corresponds to one cycle over the duration of the time series, the second lowest frequency corresponds to two cycles over the duration of the time series, and so on up to $N - 1$ cycles (where N is the number of samples in the time series). Thus, if the data time series lasts T seconds, then the sine waves that contribute to the data transform have frequencies of

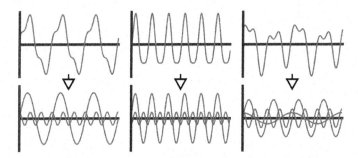

Figure 3.7 Three periodic time series (upper panels) and the corresponding sine waves (lower panels) that can be summed to create those time series.

$1/T, 2/T, 3/T, ..., (N-1)/T$ Hz. Thus, the length of the time series determines which frequencies the data is sampled at after applying the Fourier transform.

Each frequency component has two parameters which may vary: the magnitude (sometimes alternatively referred to as the amplitude), which quantifies the distance from zero of the peak of the sine wave along the amplitude axis, and the phase, which quantifies the shift of the sine wave along the time axis. Additionally, if the time series has a non-zero mean then a constant value equal to the mean must be used to fit the data in addition to the $N - 1$ sine waves. Mathematically this constant value is treated as corresponding to the 0 Hz frequency component of the data (this is sometimes called the *DC component* of the signal). Thus, once this 0 Hz is included, the data is represented by N frequencies (where again N is the number of samples in the time series). Thus, after applying the Fourier transform the data is represented by the magnitude and phase of the corresponding sine wave at each of N frequencies. This constitutes the frequency domain representation of the data. An example of this representation for a short data time series is shown in Figure 3.8.

Because of the phenomenon known as aliasing previously described in Chapter 1, frequencies above the Nyquist frequency (equal to half the sampling rate) are aliases of corresponding frequencies below the Nyquist frequency, meaning that they have equal magnitude (and phase of the opposite sign) to those frequencies. In Figure 3.8 the Nyquist frequency is labelled f_n. It can be seen that the magnitude spectrum is symmetrical around this frequency (except for the 0 Hz component) and that the phase spectrum is also symmetrical if the phase values above the Nyquist frequency are multiplied by -1. This means that magnitude and phase information for frequencies above the Nyquist frequency are redundant with those below the Nyquist frequency, and each time series can be fully represented by all frequencies up to (and including) the Nyquist frequency.

In some instances, instead of representing the signal at each frequency by values of magnitude and phase, a single, complex-valued coefficient may be used instead. A complex number is a value that is expressed in the form $a + bi$, where i is the imaginary unit, defined

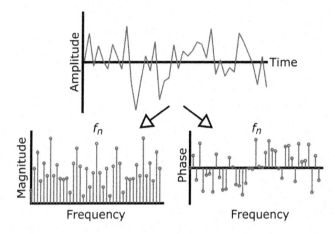

Figure 3.8 Illustration of the frequency domain representation of data. An example time series (upper panel) can be represented by measurements of magnitude (lower left panel) and phase (lower right panel) across frequency.

as being equal to the square root of -1. Each complex number therefore has two components: the first (corresponding to the value *a* in the example) is known as the *real component*, and the second (correspond to the value *b* in the example) is multiplied by *i* and is therefore known as the *imaginary component*. This complex coefficient corresponds to the fit of a complex sinusoid (a sine wave with both real and imaginary components, given by the cosine and sine functions respectively) to the data. This representation of the data contains the same information as the magnitude and phase representation: the magnitude is equal to the square root of the sum of squares of *a* and *b*, while the phase is given by applying a mathematical function known as the *2-argument arctangent* (often written as *atan2*) to the values of *b* and *a*.

The complex-valued representation of the data is more convenient for many of the mathematical operations that can be applied to frequency domain data (and therefore is frequently used in more technical parts of the MEG literature) but is less intuitive than representing the data as separate values of magnitude and phase. As this is an introductory text, we will describe the frequency (and time–frequency) representation using the concepts of magnitude and phase and will only reference the complex representation of the data where necessary.

3.3.2 The frequency domain

Analysis of MEG data in the frequency domain can be performed by applying the Fourier transform to the entire data acquisition, individual epochs or specific time windows of interest within individual epochs. Usually, the aim of the analysis is to measure the amplitude of the signal at different frequencies, or to compare the amplitude at the same frequency across conditions. Thus, most analyses focus on the magnitude rather than the phase information present in the frequency domain (we will look at phase later in Section 3.3.5).

Because the magnitude measures the distance of the peak of the corresponding sine wave along the amplitude axis, the magnitude always takes a positive value. Thus, the magnitude can be interpreted as the strength of the signal at the corresponding frequency. The distribution of magnitudes across frequencies is known as the *amplitude spectrum* (or less commonly the *frequency spectrum*). It is this spectrum that is shown for both conditions in Figure 3.6 B.

The spectrum measured from each epoch of data does not constitute an exact representation of the underlying signals (because the MEG data contains various sources of noise, and because the brain signals are inherently variable) but instead can be better considered as a noisy estimate of those signals. When treating the frequency domain representation of the data as a spectral estimate, it is common to plot the spectrum of signal *power* – which is calculated by squaring the magnitude – rather than amplitude. The distribution of power with respect to frequency is known as the *power spectrum*. The area under the power spectrum between two frequencies is proportional to the total signal power present in the data within the corresponding frequency interval (this interval is known as the *frequency band* and its width is known as the *bandwidth*). Thus, the area of the grey shaded region in Figure 3.9 gives a measure of the total signal power within

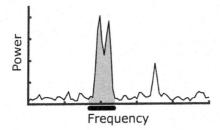

Figure 3.9 Example power spectrum. The grey shaded areas give total power in the frequency band marked by the black line below the frequency axis.

the frequency band shown by the black line (the same is not true for the amplitude spectrum which is why this is less commonly used).

The amplitude and power spectra are sampled at frequencies that contain integer numbers of cycles within the data time series (i.e. at integer multiples of $1/T$ Hz), meaning that the sampling interval of the data along the frequency axis is determined by the length of the data in the time domain. Conversely the length of the data in the frequency domain is determined by the sampling interval in the time domain. In order to maximise the frequency resolution of the spectrum the data the time series should therefore be as long as possible, whereas to maximise the range of the spectrum the sampling rate of the data time series should be as high as possible.

To sample the spectrum at a higher resolution, the data time series can be artificially lengthened by adding extra samples to the beginning and end of the time series. The amplitude of these extra samples is set to zero, and hence this process as known as *zero padding* the data. However, because this does not add any extra information to the data, it does not increase the frequency resolution of the spectrum itself, but simply alters the frequencies at which the spectrum is sampled.

In real world situations, it is rarely the case that periodic brain signals have a frequency that is exactly equal to integer multiples of $1/T$ Hz, and therefore the data is not sampled at the exact frequency of the signal. When this is the case, most of the signal power is measured at the frequency corresponding to the nearest frequency (i.e. the nearest frequency that is an integer multiple of $1/T$ Hz), but some power leaks out into other frequencies – a phenomenon known as *spectral leakage*. To reduce the effect of this leakage, it is common to multiply the time series with a window function that gradually tapers the data towards zero at the edges. This reduces the amount of leakage in the spectrum, but at the cost of introducing some smoothing of the frequency spectrum (and thus reducing the frequency resolution of the spectrum). Differing window functions may be applied to the data, each with a different trade-off between greater suppression of spectral leakage versus greater frequency resolution in the resulting spectrum.

Instead of applying a single taper function, a popular alternative approach is to apply a series of tapers to the data, known as discrete prolate spheroidal sequences (DPSS) or Slepian tapers (Thomson, 1982). This approach is known as *multitapering*. The spectrum is measured after application of each taper and then averaged across tapers. Because each taper in the sequence is designed to carry independent information about the spectrum, the process of averaging across the tapers helps to average out noise in addition to reducing spectral leakage (but at the cost of producing even greater frequency smoothing than calculating the spectrum with a single taper). This can therefore be useful in analysing data with a low signal-to-noise ratio.

3.3.3 The time–frequency domain

When analysing data in the frequency domain it is usually assumed that the data is formed from periodic signals that are stationary, that is that parameters of these signals – such as their amplitude or frequency – do not change over time (and that the statistical distribution of noise does not change over time either). However, most periodic brain signals have parameters that do vary over time and are therefore non-stationary. Such signals may be difficult to interpret and analyse based on the frequency domain representation of the data alone, because non-stationarities present in the signal are represented

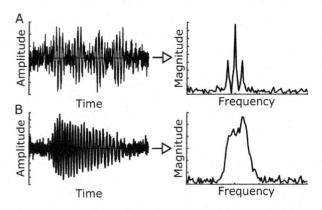

Figure 3.10 Examples of two time series containing non-stationary signals and their corresponding spectra.

by additional frequency components in the spectral representation of the data rather than as changes over time.

As an illustration, Figure 3.10 A shows data containing a periodic signal that varies in amplitude over time (plus random noise). The power spectrum of this data reveals that, in addition to the component at the frequency of the periodic signal, the varying amplitude introduces two additional frequency components. While this spectrum is an accurate representation of the data – in the sense that this reflects the sine waves that must be added together to produce the data time series – it does not really capture the fact that the data contains one periodic signal that varies in amplitude rather than three separate periodic signals. Nor would it be easy to determine the timecourse of the amplitude of the signal from the frequency domain representation. Figure 3.10 B shows an example of a signal that varies in both amplitude and frequency over time. Again, although the power spectrum gives an accurate estimate of the power present at each frequency across the whole of the time series, it is difficult to identify from the frequency domain representation that the data corresponds to a single periodic signal with time-varying amplitude and frequency.

In situations like these, the data will be better understood if analysed with respect to both frequency and time. Instead of transforming data from a representation wholly based on time to a representation wholly based on frequency, this can be achieved by creating a representation of the data based on data samples measured over both the time and frequency. Data is then said to be represented in the time–frequency domain. There are a variety of methods for calculating time–frequency representations of time series, but here we will describe a method that is an extension of the Fourier transform, known as the *short-time Fourier transform*.

To produce a representation of the data that is sampled over both time and frequency, the Fourier transform is applied not to the whole data time series, but instead to a series of shorter, overlapping time windows centred on each time sample within the series (Figure 3.11). As in the frequency domain, the windows may be

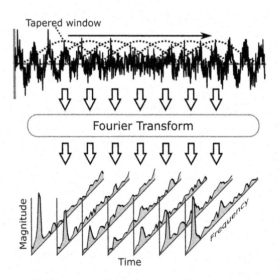

Figure 3.11   Illustration of the short-time Fourier transform. The upper panel illustrates the application of a sliding window to the data time series. Windowed data is Fourier transformed to produce a series of measurements of spectral data (lower panel) across time.

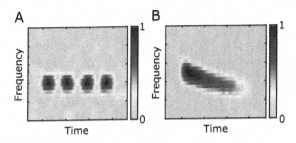

Figure 3.12 Spectrogram of the non-stationary time series shown in Figure 3.12.

tapered (or multitapered) before the Fourier transform is applied to reduce spectral leakage. Separate measures of the magnitude and phase of each frequency component can then be generated for each time window, giving a representation of the data that is sampled across both time and frequency. This corresponds to a measure of signal magnitude and phase (or the complex-valued equivalent) for each frequency at each time sample.

As in the frequency domain it is most common in the time–frequency domain to analyse the magnitude of the data. This can be plotted in the form of a *spectrogram* in which time is plotted along the x-axis, frequency along the y-axis, and signal amplitude or power is represented by the colour scale at each time–frequency sample. Figure 3.12 shows spectrograms of the time series previously shown in Figure 3.10. Power at each time–frequency sample is represented by the colour scale (because the data are in arbitrary units, each plot has been scaled so that the maximum power is equal to 1). In both plots shown in Figure 3.10 we can see how signal power at each frequency changes over time, and this illustrates how the time–frequency representation of the data can be used to measure event-related changes in periodic brain responses.

Because a separate measure of signal magnitude is calculated for each time sample in the time–frequency domain, these measures are often conceptualised as a measurement of *instantaneous magnitude* at the corresponding frequency. For periodic signals that are

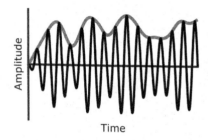

Figure 3.13 Illustration of the envelope. The envelope (grey line) reflects the time-varying amplitude of a non-stationary periodic signal (black line).

non-stationary with respect to amplitude, the variation in amplitude over time can be represented by a time series known as the *envelope* of the data (Figure 3.13). Where the aim of the analysis is to measure information about the envelope of the event-related response at a particular frequency, the time series of instantaneous amplitude or power at that frequency can be treated as the time series of the envelope of that frequency.

In addition to the short-time Fourier transform several other methods exist for converting data from the time domain to the time–frequency domain. One popular alternative is the *wavelet transform* which involves applying a mathematical process known as convolution to the data using a series of mathematical functions known as wavelets. Another alternative is to bandpass filter the data at a series of different frequency intervals and use a mathematical technique known as the *Hilbert transform* to convert the filtered data into a time series of complex coefficients. We will not discuss these alternative methods any further here as they can be shown to be formally equivalent to the short-time Fourier transform and to produce the same results provided that the parameters used for the time–frequency transform are matched across methods (Bruns, 2004). For those that are interested in exploring and comparing these methods, Part III of Cohen (2014) is recommended as an introduction to this topic.

As we noted in Section 3.3.1, the Fourier transform measures the magnitude and phase at frequencies at $1/T$ Hz intervals. In the short-time Fourier transform T corresponds to the duration of the sampling window. Thus, as the window length increases in size, the interval between frequencies decreases. The frequency resolution therefore *increases* with increasing window length. However, because neighbouring time windows of the data overlap, the Fourier transforms at each time sample will not be independent. The larger the time window, the greater the overlap between samples and therefore the greater the dependence of magnitude and phase across time samples of the time–frequency representation. Thus, the time resolution *decreases* with increasing window length.

This illustrates a fundamental trade-off that occurs for all time–frequency representations of the data (including those calculated using methods other than the short-time Fourier transform): the time and frequency resolution of the data are inversely related. This relates to the fact that, as concepts, time and frequency are themselves inversely related (i.e. frequency is equal to 1/time and vice versa). Consequently, when converting the data into the time–frequency domain there is always a trade-off in time resolution versus frequency resolution of the representation of the data. The more information the representation has about frequency (and therefore the higher the frequency resolution) the less it has about time (and therefore the lower the time resolution) and vice versa. By varying the window length (and the function used for tapering) it is possible to create a range of time–frequency representations of the data with different levels of trade-off between time and frequency resolution. Therefore, when calculating a time–frequency representation of the data, the user must decide what compromise they wish to make between time and frequency resolution.

One final point of note relates to the length, rather than resolution, of the time component of the time–frequency representation. For samples close to the edge of the time series the corresponding window will extend outside of the data. This means these time samples will not be included in the time–frequency representation. To avoid this, the time–frequency representation must be calculated from a longer time series or, if this is not possible, some form of data padding must be used to extend the length of the time series (although note that padding will generally introduce data artefacts at the edges of the data).

3.3.4 Data analysis in the frequency and time–frequency domains

Once data has been transformed into the frequency and time–frequency domains, the aim is typically to measure an event-related response of some kind. However, as we have already seen when looking at the time domain, MEG is inherently noisy and averaging data across epochs is necessary to average out noise and reveal event-related responses. Thus, when analysing data based on measures of amplitude or power in the frequency or time–frequency domains it is usually also necessary to average data across epochs. However, there are two separate ways the data can be averaged, each with their own advantages.

Firstly, as we have seen in the previous section, averaging data in the time domain preserves event-related signals while reducing signals (including noise signals) that are not time-locked to the experimental event. Therefore, if data is first averaged in the time domain before being converted into the frequency or time–frequency domains, the presence of non-event-related signals should be attenuated in the data (due to having been averaged out) while event-related signals should be unaffected. The magnitude data will therefore primarily reflect signals time-locked to the experimental event (plus some residual contribution of non-time-locked signals that have not completely averaged out).

However, there are many brain signals that show event-related changes in signal power, but where the phase of the signal is not consistent across epochs. Although the change in power is time-locked to the experimental event, the difference in phase across epochs means that the signal itself is not time-locked to the event. A disadvantage of averaging the data in the time domain is that these signals tend to average out, and only those responses that are *phase-locked* (as well as time-locked) to the event will be retained in the averaged data.

In order to measure responses that are not phase-locked, data for each epoch must first be converted to the frequency or time–frequency domain, and measures of amplitude or power averaged across epochs. Because information about phase is not included when averaging across epochs, the averaged spectra will still contain brain signals that are not phase-locked to the experimental event. However, the disadvantage of this approach is that other signals that are not phase-locked to the experimental event, such as noise signals, are no longer averaged out either. The spectrum or spectrogram will measure all signals present in the data, not just those that are event-related, and additional processing of the data is required to eliminate the contribution of signals that are not event-related. Typically, this is achieved by applying baseline correction to the data. Signals that are not event-related (including noise signals) should be present in a baseline time period, and therefore subtracting a corresponding measure of baseline amplitude or power from the data should subtract out these non-event-related signals.

In summary, data can be averaged first in the time domain before converting to the frequency and time–frequency domains. This reduces the contribution of signals that are not event-related, but at the expense of also reducing event-related responses that are not phase-locked to the experimental event. Alternatively, data can be converted to the frequency and time–frequency domains and the magnitudes averaged across epochs. In this case non-phase-locked responses are preserved in the average but signals that are not event-related are not reduced and need to be removed by other means (typically by performing baseline correction).

Once the data has been averaged and baseline corrected then similar analysis methods can be applied as in the time domain. Data can be contrasted across conditions either for each frequency or time–frequency sample, or for components of the response occurring within specific frequency bands or time–frequency windows. We will look in more detail at how statistical comparisons are performed on MEG data in Chapter 4.

3.3.5 Phase

Although we have focused so far on the analysis of magnitude, data in the frequency and time–frequency domains is also represented by phase. The phase of each frequency component represents the shift of the corresponding sine wave along the time axis, as illustrated in Figure 3.14. When phase is measured using the Fourier transform, the phase is 0° when the peaks of the sine wave occur at the start and end of the time window (i.e. where the time series matches a cosine function) and other phases are measured relative to this: rightward and leftward shifts correspond to decreases and increases of phase, respectively.

Phase is measured on a circular scale and is therefore represented by an angle (as shown by the circles in Figure 3.14). The use of a circular scale captures the fact that a shift along the time axis through

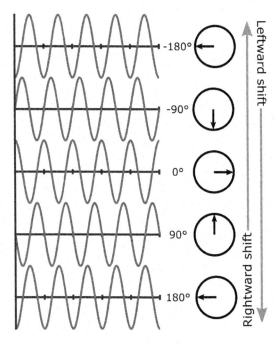

Figure 3.14 Illustration of the concept of phase. The position of the sine wave along the time axis can be represented by a corresponding angular quantity.

one whole cycle leaves the sine wave unchanged (this can be seen by comparing the top and bottom panels of Figure 3.10), just as one full rotation around a circle leaves the angle unchanged. Because of this circular property, phase is often constrained to be between -180° and 180° (or alternatively between 0° and 360°), as values of phase outside this range are identical to corresponding vales inside the range (e.g. a phase of 270° is identical to a phase of -90°).

In general, data analysis in the frequency domain tends to focus on magnitude rather than phase, because experimental hypotheses more commonly relate to differences in the strength of periodic signals, rather than on the position of the waveform along the time axis. The fact that phase is represented on a circular scale also presents technical challenges because most descriptive statistics and statistical tests are not designed for use with angular quantities and therefore are unsuitable for analysis of phase. For instance, the mean of 20 and 350 is 185, but the mean of 20° and 350° angles is 15° (this corresponds to a quantity known as the circular mean). Thus, statistical analysis of phase must be performed using statistical techniques specifically designed for circular variables.

As discussed in Section 3.3.4 some event-related responses have a consistent phase across epochs and are therefore said to be phase-locked to the event, while other responses show variability in their phase across epochs. Because of this, the most common analyses of phase in the frequency domain involve measurements of the consistency of phase across epochs to detect the presence of phase-locking. This is measured using a quantity – which we will refer to here as *phase coherence* but which is also known by other names such *phase synchrony, phase-locking value, phase-locking factor* or *inter-trial phase clustering* – that measures the consistency of the phase across epochs on a scale between zero (indicating no consistency across epochs) and one (indicating perfect consistency across epochs) (Lachaux et al., 1999; Mormann et al., 2000). Thus, unlike phase itself, phase coherence is not represented on a circular scale. Phase coherence can be measured at a single frequency of interest or can be measured for each frequency to produce a phase coherence spectrum.

When working in the time–frequency domain, phase represents which part of the sine wave is present at the current time sample

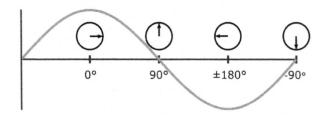

Figure 3.15 Illustration of instantaneous phase at four time points within a single cycle of a sine wave.

(Figure 3.15). This is sometimes called the *instantaneous phase*. As with measurements of phase in the frequency domain, the most common use of instantaneous phase is to measure phase coherence of the data across epochs, but with the advantage that this can be measured across time as well as frequency, so that the timecourse of phase coherence can be analysed.

When combined with measures of instantaneous magnitude, instantaneous phase can also be used to measure a phenomenon known as *cross-frequency coupling*. This is where the instantaneous phase or amplitude at one frequency varies with respect to the instantaneous phase or amplitude of another frequency. This most commonly takes the form of phase-amplitude coupling in which the amplitude envelope at one frequency varies with the instantaneous phase at a second (usually lower) frequency. For more information about cross-frequency coupling and how it is measured, see Canolty & Knight, (2010).

3.3.6 Summary

In this section we have seen that MEG data time series can be transformed into representations of the data as a series of measures (magnitude and phase) over frequency, or over both time and frequency. These correspond to the frequency domain and time–frequency domain representation of the data, respectively. The frequency domain representation is particularly useful for analysing periodic brain responses present in the data, especially if their parameters are unchanging within each epoch (in which case the signals are said to be stationary). Conversely, the time–frequency domain is useful for measuring periodic responses whose parameters vary over time (that is, responses that are non-stationary).

Further reading

Burgess, R. C. (2020). Recognizing and correcting MEG artifacts. *Journal of Clinical Neurophysiology, 37*(6), 508–517. https://doi.org/10.1097/WNP.0000000000000699

Cohen, M. X. (2014). *Analyzing neural time series data: Theory and practice.* MIT Press. https://doi.org/10.7551/mitpress/9609.001.0001

de Cheveigné, A., & Nelken, I. (2019). Filters: When, why, and how (not) to use them. *Neuron, 102*(2), 280–293. https://doi.org/10.1016/J.NEURON.2019.02.039

Hari, R., & Puce, A. (2017). *MEG-EEG Primer.* Oxford University Press. https://doi.org/10.1093/med/9780190497774.001.0001

Keil, A., et al. (2022). Recommendations and publication guidelines for studies using frequency domain and time-frequency domain analyses of neural time series. *Psychophysiology, 59*(5), e14502. https://doi.org/10.1111/psyp.14052

Luck, S. J. (2014). *An introduction to the event-related potential technique.* MIT Press. https://mitpress.ublish.com/book/introduction-event-related-potential-technique-0

References

Acunzo, D. J., MacKenzie, G., & van Rossum, M. C. W. (2012). Systematic biases in early ERP and ERF components as a result of high-pass filtering. *Journal of Neuroscience Methods, 209*(1), 212–218. https://doi.org/10.1016/J.JNEUMETH.2012.06.011

Bruns, A. (2004). Fourier-, Hilbert-and wavelet-based signal analysis: are they really different approaches? *Journal of Neuroscience Methods, 137*, 321–332. https://doi.org/10.1016/j.jneumeth.2004.03.002

Canolty, R. T., & Knight, R. T. (2010). The functional role of cross-frequency coupling. *Trends in Cognitive Sciences, 14*(11), 506–515. https://doi.org/10.1016/j.tics.2010.09.001

Cohen, M. X. (2014). *Analyzing Neural Time Series Data: Theory and Practice.* MIT Press. https://doi.org/10.7551/mitpress/9609.001.0001

de Cheveigné, A., & Nelken, I. (2019). Filters: When, why, and how (not) to use them. *Neuron, 102*(2), 280–293. https://doi.org/10.1016/J.NEURON.2019.02.039

Gratton, G., Coles, M. G. H., & Donchin, E. (1983). A new method for off-line removal of ocular artifact. *Electroencephalography and Clinical Neurophysiology, 55*(4). https://doi.org/10.1016/0013-4694(83)90135-9

Groppe, D. M., Urbach, T. P., & Kutas, M. (2011). Mass univariate analysis of event-related brain potentials/fields I: A critical tutorial review. *Psychophysiology, 48*(12), 1711. https://doi.org/10.1111/J.1469-8986.2011.01273.X

Ikeda, S., & Toyama, K. (2000). Independent component analysis for noisy data – MEG data analysis. *Neural Networks, 13*(10). https://doi.org/10.1016/S0893-6080(00)00071-X

Kappenman, E. S., & Luck, S. J. (2012). *The Oxford Handbook of Event-related Potential Components.* Oxford University Press. https://doi.org/10.1093/oxfordhb/9780195374148.001.0001

Lachaux, J. P., Rodriguez, E., Martinerie, J., & Varela, F. J. (1999). Measuring phase synchrony in brain signals. *Human Brain Mapping, 8*(4), 194. https://doi.org/10.1002/(sici)1097-0193(1999)8:4<194::aid-hbm4>3.0.co;2-c

Luck, S. J. (2014). *An Introduction to the Event-Related Potential Technique, second edition.* The MIT Press.

Mormann, F., Lehnertz, K., David, P., & Elger, C. E. (2000). Mean phase coherence as a measure for phase synchronization and its application to the EEG of epilepsy patients. *Physica D: Nonlinear Phenomena, 144*(3–4), 358–369. https://doi.org/10.1016/S0167-2789(00)00087-7

Taulu, S., Kajola, M., & Simola, J. (2004). Suppression of interference and artifacts by the signal space separation method. *Brain Topography, 16*(4). https://doi.org/10.1023/B:BRAT.0000032864.93890.f9

Thomson, D. J. (1982). Spectrum estimation and harmonic analysis. *Proceedings of the IEEE, 70*(9). https://doi.org/10.1109/PROC.1982.12433

Uusitalo, M. A., & Ilmoniemi, R. J. (1997). Signal-space projection method for separating MEG or EEG into components. *Medical and Biological Engineering and Computing, 35*(2). https://doi.org/10.1007/BF02534144

Chapter 4

Analysing spatial information

In the previous chapter we looked how individual data time series can be analysed. However, in practice it is unusual to analyse data based on a single MEG sensor. Instead, it is more common to use information about the distribution of the magnetic field across the sensor array to make inferences about the location, as well as timing, of brain responses. Thus, in this chapter we will look at how spatial information present in the data can be analysed and interpreted.

Whereas MEG has a high temporal resolution that provides a rich level of information about temporal aspects of the brain's signals, it has a relatively low spatial resolution compared to other techniques for non-invasive imaging of the brain (particularly fMRI). Despite this, useful information about the spatial location of the source currents that generate the brain's magnetic field can be still derived from MEG data. This information can be analysed in two alternative ways: by measuring the spatial pattern of the magnetic field across the sensor array, or by estimating the spatial location of the sources themselves within the brain. These correspond to *sensor space* and *source space* representations of the data, respectively. In the first two sections of this chapter we will look at how these two representations of the data can be used to spatially localise the brain signals present in the MEG data. Then in the third and final section we will explore how statistical hypothesis testing can be applied to the data.

DOI: 10.4324/9781315205175-6

4.1 Sensor space

4.1.1 Interpreting the spatial distribution of the magnetic field

At each time sample, MEG data is represented by a measurement at each sensor. However, the magnetic field of each individual source is not restricted to an individual sensor but instead spreads out across the whole sensor array. This phenomenon is often referred to as *field spread*. Thus, localisation of brain responses must be achieved by analysing the spatial pattern of the magnetic field across sensors, rather than based on the measurement at individual sensors.

To illustrate this, Figure 4.1 shows examples of the magnetic field measurements made by each of the three different types of sensor

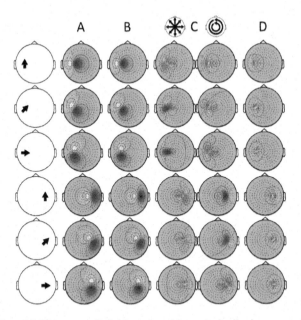

Figure 4.1 The magnetic field produced by a single dipolar source in different positions and orientations measured using magnetometers (A), axial gradiometers (B), pairs of planar gradiometers (C) and combined planar gradiometers (D).

from a single dipolar source at two positions and three orientations. We can see that the spatial pattern of the magnetic field varies in predictable ways that can provide information about the position and orientation of the source current.

Because magnetometers and axial gradiometers (shown in Figure 4.1 A and 4.1B respectively) measure the magnetic field strength/gradient in the same direction, they measure a similar spatial pattern for dipolar sources, with the main difference being that the field gradient decreases more rapidly with distance from the source, meaning that the field spread is reduced for gradiometers relative to magnetometers. Both types of sensor exhibit a distinct pattern of measurements for a dipolar source. The sensors that have the largest amplitude are not those directly over the source. Instead, the measurements are strongest where the magnetic field is oriented perpendicular to the surface of the head. This occurs at two locations on either side of the source. The fields either side of the source also have opposite signs, reflecting the fact the measured field is exiting the head on one side of the source and entering on the other.

Thus, when measured with magnetometers or axial gradiometers, the spatial pattern of the field measurements must be interpreted in a specific way: the position of the source lies between the sensors with largest positive and negative amplitudes while the orientation of the source is at a 90° clockwise rotation from a line connecting these sensors. This can make sensor space analysis of magnetometers and axial gradiometer data complicated because the magnetic field generated by each source is not restricted to a single contiguous region of the sensor array. Thus, statistical analysis of the data shown in Figure 4.1 would reveal two discrete clusters of sensors that are significantly different from zero when in fact the data corresponds to a single source.

To further complicate matters, measurements made by planar gradiometers have a different spatial pattern to this and therefore must be interpreted differently. As mentioned in Chapter 1, planar gradiometers are generally arranged in pairs of sensors oriented at 90° from each other. Thus, Figure 4.1 C shows two plots, each corresponding to one of the two directions in which the field is measured (gradiometers in the first column are oriented away from the centre of the sensor array and those in the second column are oriented 90° anti-clockwise to the corresponding sensor in the first column). In contrast to the other two sensor types the strongest response is found at the sensor location closest to the dipolar source, but the relative amplitude measured at each sensor within each pair depends on the orientation of the source relative to the sensors. This makes it difficult to measure the strength of the source in an orientation independent way.

To deal with this issue, the measurements made by planar gradiometers are usually combined across each pair of sensors by calculating the square root of the sum of squares of each data sample across the sensor pair (or in the frequency or time-frequency domains, the square root of the sum of the squared magnitudes). Examples of this combined planar data are shown in the last column of Figure 4.1 D. In the combined planar representation of the data, the sensors with the largest magnitude form a single cluster, with the sensor directly over the source having the largest amplitude. This makes it easier to infer the location of the underlying sources from the sensor space data, as well as making the data more suited for cluster-based statistical analysis (see Section 4.3.3). For this reason, researchers using data collected from magnetometers or axial gradiometers may also sometimes transform the data to a representation of the planar gradient (this can be achieved by calculating the spatial derivative of the data).

Note, however, that because the combined gradient only takes positive values, information about the direction of the source current (which is carried by the sign of the magnetic field) is lost after combing the gradiometers. The loss of the sign of the field also means that it is necessary to perform processing steps such as filtering, averaging and transformation into the frequency or time–frequency domains before combining each gradiometer pair.

So far, we have seen that the position and orientation of a source relative to the two-dimensional surface of the sensor array can be inferred from the data, provided the pattern of field measurements expected for each sensor type is known. However, the depth of the source within the head is more difficult to determine due to an inherent ambiguity between source depth and extent.

Figure 4.2 illustrates the measurements for a dipolar source at two different depths and shows that, where data is generated by

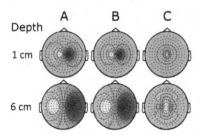

Figure 4.2 The magnetic field produced by a single dipolar source at two different depths measured using magnetometers (A), axial gradiometers (B), and combined planar gradiometers (C).

a single dipolar source, the field spread increases with increasing source depth. Thus, assuming a single dipolar source, information about the depth of the source can be inferred from the field spread (for magnetometers and axial gradiometers, the depth should be approximately proportional to the distance between the maximum and minimum field measurements). However, field spread also increases when the spatial spread of the source current increases, and thus deep, focal sources and shallow, extended sources may produce similar (or even identical) fields, making it difficult to distinguish between them. For this reason, information about source depth can be ambiguous if information about the strength or spatial extent of the source currents is unknown.

So far, we have considered the sensor measurements we would expect to see when there is only a single dipolar source. How can data be interpreted where there are multiple dipolar sources? As we learned in Chapter 1, the magnetic field produced by multiple dipoles is simply the sum of the fields produced by the individual dipoles. Thus, the spatial pattern of the magnetic field across the sensor array for multiple sources will be the sum of the spatial patterns made by the individual sources. Because the magnetic field is not limited to individual sensors and exhibits field spread this means that, where multiple sources are present, the measurement made at each sensor is a mixture of the magnetic fields generated by each of the sources.

Where there are a small number of sources with limited field spread that are distantly spaced within the brain, the fields generated by the sources will tend to be non-overlapping. This means responses generated by the different sources can be analysed separately by simply analysing the data from different sensors. However, where the magnetic fields from each source show greater levels of overlap (either due to being close together or exhibiting large field spread) then the magnetic field measurements made at each sensor reflect a mixture of the different sources. This makes it difficult to determine the contribution of each source to each sensor. A further problem is caused by the fact that the fields of different sources will tend to cancel when they overlap and are oriented in opposite directions. This field cancellation will lead to the loss of some information about the underlying source distribution.

Difficulties with analysing data in sensor space also arise from the fact that the MEG sensors are not fixed relative to the head, and therefore the position of the sensors relative to the head will vary across participants. This means that the position and spread of the magnetic field may vary across subjects, or across different sessions with the same subject, even when the source location itself does not vary.

In conclusion, although analysis in sensor space is the most straight forward approach, these are specific issues that limit its usefulness in localising brain activity. Provided that the relationship between sources and the corresponding field pattern measured by the sensors is understood, then sensor space analysis can be a useful way to analyse data generated by either a single source or a small number of sources with largely non-overlapping magnetic fields. However, where data is generated by a more complex source distribution, it is difficult to separate the contribution of each source to the magnetic field when working in sensor space. In this circumstance it will generally be easier to interpret and analyse the data in source space.

4.1.2 Summary

In this section we have seen that MEG data can be analysed with respect to the spatial distribution of the magnetic field across the sensors. This is known as analysing the data in sensor space.

When working in sensor space the spatial distribution of the magnetic field contains information about the location of the underlying source currents. In order to accurately interpret this information from MEG data it is necessary to understand the magnetic field measurements made by the specific sensor type (magnetometers, axial gradiometers, or planar gradiometers) in the presence of source currents. However, the information present in the source space representation of the data is ambiguous with respect to information such as the depth and number of sources and may be difficult to interpret, especially where several sources are present simultaneously. Therefore, sensors space analyses may be best suited to situations in which there is known to be a small number of sources that have non-overlapping magnetic fields.

4.2 Source space

Rather than analyse data based on the spatial pattern of the magnetic field across sensors, it is instead possible to estimate the distribution of source currents that generated the magnetic field. It is this approach that forms the basis of analysis in source space.

However, there is no single method that is guaranteed to produce an accurate estimation of the sources in all circumstances. Any magnetic field measured at the sensors is consistent with more than one possible configuration of source currents and therefore it is not possible to unambiguously determine the sources of the brain's magnetic field if no additional information about those sources is known (or can be assumed).

In this section, we will first look at why this problem exists and what its implications are for MEG source analysis. We will follow this by looking at the techniques that can be used to solve this problem and enable MEG data to be analysed in source space.

4.2.1 The MEG inverse problem

Often in science we may have some knowledge of the current state of a physical system and wish to predict what measurements we would expect to make given that state. In the context of MEG this would correspond to knowing the current state of the brain's electrical currents and predicting what magnetic field measurements we would expect to make at each of the sensors. Such problems are known as *forward problems,* because they involve calculating forward from a mathematical model of a physical system to a set of predicted observations. In other circumstances, we may start with a set of measurements which we wish to use to infer the current state of the system that gave rise to those measurements. Such problems are known as *inverse problems,* because they involve working backward from a set of observations to find a model (and a set of model parameters) that account for those observations. Inferring the sources of the brain's magnetic field is a problem that involves using the measurements of the magnetic field outside of the head to estimate a model of the source currents that produced those observations, and thus is a type of inverse problem. For this reason, the methods used for solving this problem by estimating the sources of the magnetic fields are often called *inverse methods.*

One issue with solving inverse problems is that they are often *ill-posed,* meaning that there is no unique solution to the problem. This is the case for the MEG inverse problem, due to the fact that any magnetic field measured outside of the head can be explained by many different sets of sources (infinitely many in theory), with no way to determine which is the correct source configuration based on the data alone. This is because it is not possible to determine the distribution of current within a conductive volume (such as the head) based on measurements made from outside of the volume (such as the magnetic field measurements made outside of the head).

This would seem to imply that it is impossible to accurately estimate the sources of the magnetic field measured outside of the head, which would make it impossible to analyse MEG data in source space. However, although we cannot constrain the MEG inverse problem to a unique solution based on the data alone, if we are willing to make some assumptions about the source distribution then it becomes possible to restrict the inverse problem to a single, unique solution. However, this estimate of the source distribution will only be accurate to the extent that these assumptions are correct.

This means that there is no single 'correct' method for MEG source estimation that is guaranteed to be accurate in all situations. Instead, there are multiple methods available for source estimation of MEG data, each applying different assumptions about the sources. Here we will explore some of the more commonly used of these methods.

4.2.2 The forward problem

All solutions to the MEG inverse problem require us to first understand what observations we should expect given a set of source currents present in the brain. Thus, all MEG inverse solutions require us to first solve the MEG forward problem. To achieve this, we must first produce an accurate *forward model* of the magnetic field generated outside of the head for each possible configuration of source currents. This allows us to calculate the magnetic field that would be generated by different sources in the brain (for instance, all the field measurements shown in Figures 4.1 and 4.2 were calculated using a forward model) and this information can be used in the calculation of the inverse solution.

There are two components of MEG forward models. The first component is the *source model*: a mathematical model of the source currents and their associated magnetic field is required. As we encountered in Chapter 1, impressed current flowing synchronously within a local population of neurons can generally be well approximated by a source of infinitesimal extent known as an equivalent current dipole. The current dipole therefore forms the source model in almost all MEG forward models. Each dipolar source can be characterised by just six parameters: three location parameters defining the position of the dipole in the three dimensions of space, two orientation parameters (in a spherical coordinate system these typically will correspond to angle of the dipole from the radial axis and the angle of the dipole in the tangential plane) and the dipole moment (alternatively, the dipole moment and orientation may be represented by a vector defining the moment in three dimensions). Because the magnetic field of dipoles combines additively across sources, it is only necessary to calculate the forward model for all possible parameters of a single source, as the magnetic field generated by multiple sources can be calculated as the sum of the field generated by the individual sources.

The second component of the forward model is the *head model*: a mathematical model of the conductive properties of the head. This is a necessary component of the forward model because, as we have seen in Chapter 1, the magnetic field measured outside the head is dependent on the volume current as well as the impressed current. We must therefore model the current flow throughout the volume of the head in order to understand how the volume currents contribute to the magnetic field measurements. To achieve this, it is necessary to produce a model of the head in which the different biological tissues (e.g. brain, skull, scalp) are treated as a series of nested volumes where each volume may be defined by both its shape and conductance.

It is necessary to know the position of the brain surface (and/or the surface of other tissues such as the skull and scalp) relative to the MEG sensors to produce an accurate head model. The is normally achieved by identifying the position of the head localisation coils on the subject's structural MRI (or on a surrogate MRI, if the subject's own image is not available), a process known as *coregistration*. The most common approach to coregistering the coils to the MRI is to use a 3D digitiser at the time of data acquisition to acquire a representation of the subject's scalp surface and the position of the coils relative to that surface. By fitting the digitised scalp surface to the MRI scalp surface, this gives the position of the coils within the MRI, which in turn gives the position of the brain and other head structures relative to the sensors. The brain, scalp and other surfaces can then be extracted from the MRI in order to create the head model.

There are two broad classes of models that are used to model the volume currents: analytical models in which the relationship between the source parameters and the predicted magnetic field are expressed in one or more equations that allow the predicted field to be calculated directly, and numerical models in which the magnetic field produced by the volume currents must be calculated using computer simulation of current flow within the head.

We have already covered the simplest analytical model of the head in Chapter 1, when we looked at the magnetic field produced when the brain is modelled as a spherical volume conductor. An important result in MEG forward modelling is that if we treat the head tissues (e.g. brain, skull, scalp) as set of spherical volumes, the magnetic field produced outside the head is independent of the diameter or electrical conductivity of any of the individual volumes (Sarvas, 1987). This means the forward model is independent of the number of spheres or their individual properties and can instead be modelled as a single sphere of unspecified conductance. The effects of the volume currents no longer need to be explicitly modelled but can be included in the model by making an appropriate adjustment to the equation used to calculate the magnetic field of the current dipole (in this case, the number of parameters of the dipole is reduced from six to five as the radial component of the moment does not contribute to the external magnetic field).

Because of its simplicity the spherical head model is the most commonly used in MEG forward modelling. The head model can be created for each subject by fitting a sphere to either the brain or scalp surface extracted from the coregistered MRI. However, the head is not strictly spherical, so the forward model based on a spherical head will only be approximately accurate. One adjustment of the model that has been found to improve accuracy is to use multiple overlapping spheres rather than a single sphere (Huang et al., 1999). In this case, a separate sphere is fit for each sensor based on the section of the surface closest to the sensor and the forward model for each sensor is then calculated from the corresponding sphere. Another approach is to use a mathematical technique known as spherical harmonics to model the brain as a single volume with a smoothly curving, but non-spherical, surface (Nolte, 2003). This is often known as a *single shell* model.

In order for the relationship between source current and the predicted magnetic field to be described by a single equation (or set of equations), analytical models (such as those described above) require head volumes to have a simple geometry. More accurate head models with more realistic geometry require the use of numerical methods. One such approach is to assume that the head is formed from several non-spherical volumes of homogeneous and isotropic conductance. In this case the magnetic field due to the volume currents is determined by the voltage across the boundaries between the volumes. These tissue boundaries can be extracted from the subject's coregistered MRI and represented as a series of meshes. A technique called the *boundary element method* (BEM) can then be used to compute the volume currents (and their contribution to the external magnetic field) by simulating the voltage across each point within each mesh (Fuchs et al., 2002; Oostendorp & Van Oosterom, 1989).

Alternatively, if the tissues are assumed to have inhomogeneous and/or anisotropic conductance, then a technique called the *finite element method* (FEM) can be used (Vorwerk et al., 2014). This involves dividing the entire head volume (rather than just the boundaries) into a mesh, assigning a separate conductivity to each point in the mesh, then simulating the flow of volume current through the mesh in order to calculate the predicted magnetic field.

However, numerical models – such as those based on boundary element and finite element methods – tend to require a much larger set of calculations than analytical methods, and therefore can be highly computationally intensive and time-consuming to run. Therefore, while numerical methods are commonly used for EEG forward modelling (due to the strong influence of the conductive properties of the head on the scalp potentials), analytical methods, such as the spherical and single-shell methods described above, are much more frequently used for forward modelling of MEG data.

Once a particular head model has been selected it is then possible to calculate a forward model of the MEG signal. This is generally represented by the *lead field*, which gives the sensitivity of each sensor to each possible source location in the brain. Where the orientation of each source is fixed, the lead field corresponds to a matrix that maps the sensitivity of each sensor to a source of unit moment at each location in the head. Where the orientation of the sources may vary, then the lead field of each sensor is represented by a series of vectors, where each value in the vector gives the sensitivity of the sensor when the corresponding source is oriented in each of the three dimensions of space.

Once the forward model has been created, it is then possible to calculate what measurements would be produced by a hypothetical source of known parameters (i.e. position, orientation, and moment). This information is used when calculating the solution to the MEG inverse problem, as any solution must be consistent with the forward model. However, the forward model itself does not provide a unique solution to the inverse problem. Instead, to estimate the sources of the magnetic field we must apply additional assumptions to constrain the source distribution to a single, unique solution. There are a variety of methods used for achieving this, but most are variations on two basic approaches: model fitting and spatial filtering.

4.2.3 Inverse solutions: model fitting

Some of the most widely used techniques solving the MEG inverse problem work by specifying a model of the underlying source distribution and performing a fitting procedure to find the set of model parameters that best fits the data. In this section we will look at some of these approaches.

One approach is to assume that the MEG measurements can be explained by a small number of equivalent current dipoles (Mosher et al., 1992). As each dipole has just six parameters (or five parameters when using a spherical head model) the use of a small number of dipoles means that there are fewer source parameters than there are sensor measurements. This ensures that there is a uniquely best fitting set of source parameters that explains the data and the inverse problem can therefore be solved by finding these parameters. This can be achieved setting the dipole parameters based on an initial 'best guess' and then using a fitting procedure to iteratively adjust the parameters to maximise the goodness of fit between the magnetic field that would be generated by the sources (calculated using the forward model) and the measured field. This is illustrated in Figure 4.3, where the position, orientation and moment of a single dipolar source is varied iteratively in order to match the predicted field to a measured field (shown on the right of the figure). The best fitting set of dipole parameters correspond to the estimate of the source(s) of the magnetic field. This is the oldest method of MEG source estimation and is known as *dipole fitting*.

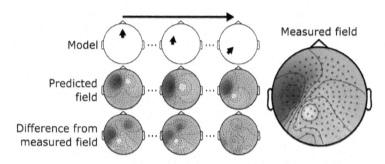

Figure 4.3 Illustration of steps in an iterative dipole fitting process when used to fit a single dipolar source to the field shown on the right.

A separate fit can be performed for each time sample, allowing the position and orientation of each dipole to change over time. The source solution then corresponds to a series of locations, orientations and moments that vary over time for each dipole. This is often known as a *moving dipole* fit. Alternatively, it may be plausible to assume that position and orientation of each source is fixed within a time window of interest, in which case the best fitting location and orientation of the dipolar sources can be found across all time samples within the time window, with only the dipole moment varying across samples. This is often known as a *fixed dipole* or *spatiotemporal* fit. Each dipole is then represented by a time series of moment that can be analysed with the techniques described in Chapter 3.

Dipole fitting methods are best suited to situations in which the magnetic field can be characterised by a relatively small number of sources. As the number of dipoles used in the model increases, the greater the likelihood that the procedure will become trapped in a local minimum of the search space (in non-technical terms, this means that the fitting procedure will converge on a solution which is a better fit then other similar solutions, but which does not correspond to the best fit overall). This means that the solution found by the fitting procedure will become increasingly dependent on the initial parameters used to perform the fit and will not always be guaranteed to be the overall best fitting solution. Dipole fitting methods are therefore best suited to situations where a small number of focal sources are present, for instance, when measuring sensory responses that can be modelled by a dipolar source (or sources) in the corresponding sensory cortices or focal epileptic discharges which are well represented by a single dipolar source (we will look at examples of both in the next chapter). In order to perform a dipole fit it is also necessary to pre-specify the number of sources to be included, and therefore the technique generally can only be used where the number of sources is already known or at least can be reasonably guessed.

Where a larger number of sources are thought to be present or where the number of sources is unknown and cannot be reasonably estimated then rather than perform an iterative fit a scanning method can be used, in which the fitting procedure scans through a set of predefined locations (such as on a regular grid within the brain volume) in order to determine the best fitting source parameters. The *multiple signal classification* (MUSIC) family of methods are an example of this approach (Mosher et al., 1992).

In many circumstances the brain's magnetic field is not generated by a small number of sources, but instead by a large number of sources widely distributed across the brain. Thus, MEG researchers have increasingly turned away from dipole fitting towards methods based on fitting the magnetic field to a dense grid of dipolar sources at fixed locations across the brain. Typically, the sources are constrained to the cortical surface (with source orientation sometimes constrained to be perpendicular to the surface) extracted from the subject's structural MRI so that the source solution can be treated as a 2D surface map of source current density. The source solution can then be found by simultaneously fitting the dipole moments of all these sources to the measured magnetic field. However, because the number of sources exceeds the number of sensors, the number of model parameters is far larger than the number of sensors. This means that many different source solutions will fit the data perfectly, and it is therefore necessary to apply additional constraints to the source estimation in order to produce a unique solution.

There are many different constraints that have been proposed to constrain distributed source solutions, and many different approaches to finding the best fitting sources solution based on those constraints, but by far the most frequently used approach is based on a method known as *minimum norm estimation* (MNE) (Hämäläinen & Ilmoniemi, 1994). This technique constrains the inverse solution to be the source estimate that minimises the total power (i.e. the sum of squared dipole moments) of the sources. Solutions that minimise source power are favoured because the least-squares best fit of the source parameters can be calculated directly from the lead field and a measurement of the noise covariance (which can be estimated from a baseline time window). This means that, in contrast to dipole fitting, it is unnecessary to perform a time-consuming fitting process to estimate the source distribution.

The source solutions produced by minimum norm estimation tend to be highly distributed, as source power can be minimised by fitting the measured magnetic field with many dipoles each of relatively small moment, rather than a small number of sources with large moment. Thus, this approach to solving the inverse problem tends to work best when the measured magnetic field was produced by a distributed (rather than focal) set of source currents.

To illustrate this, Figure 4.4 shows the event-related response of a single subject to presentation of written sentences averaged over time within four time intervals (data is taken from the study of Wang

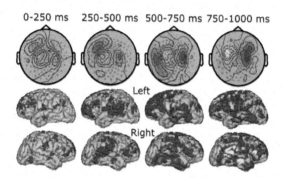

Figure 4.4 Sensor space data for four time intervals following presentation of a written sentence and the corresponding minimum norm estimation of the source distribution.

et al., 2012). Data is plotted both in source space and in sensor space following minimum norm estimation. Whereas the source solutions produced by dipole fitting methods described earlier correspond to a small number of point sources, here we can see that minimum norm estimation produces a source solution that contains activity much more widely distributed across the cortex.

One weakness of minimum norm estimation is that it introduces a depth bias to the source solution. As discussed in Section 4.2.1, the magnetic field of a deep, focal source can be identical to a shallower, extended source. Because the shallower source is more spatially distributed, it can be fit by dipoles with less total power than the deeper source, and thus minimum norm solutions are biased in favour of shallow sources that are closer to the sensors. One solution to this problem is to weight source power inversely to depth, and to calculate the source solution that minimises depth-weighted power (this is often known as *weighted minimum norm estimation* or wMNE) (Jeffs et al., 1987). Alternatively, source power can be scaled by a projection of noise power at the same location (this is known as *noise normalisation*). Because the projection of noise power is subject to the same depth bias as the source power, this scaling leads to the depth bias being divided out of the power of each source. Two methods are widely used for this calculation: *dynamic statistical parametric mapping* (dSPM) (Dale et al., 2000) and *standardised low resolution brain electromagnetic tomography* (sLORETA) (Pascual-Marqui, 2002) – each uses a different estimate of noise variance.

When interpreting source maps produced by minimum norm estimation (or by other distributed source models) it is important to be aware of a fundamental limitation on the ability of the fitting method to separate out sources mixed at the sensor level. As discussed in Section 4.2.1, where multiple sources are present the magnetic field measurements made at each sensor reflect a mixture of the fields generated by each source. Ideally, we would wish the model fit to be able to separate the contribution of each source to the data. In practice, because there are a much larger number of sources than sensors, it is not possible for the source estimates to be fully independent from each other. The consequence of this is that signal will 'leak' from the location of a true source to other locations with a similar lead field (this is sometimes known as *signal leakage* or *source leakage*). Thus, for minimum norm estimation (and for other methods for estimating distributed sources) there is a limit to the extent that brain signals which are mixed in sensor space can be unmixed at the source level.

Distributed source solutions such as minimum norm estimation are best suited to situations where source currents are distributed very widely across the brain. Because distributed source modelling necessarily favours distributed source solutions, sources will always tend to have a large spatial spread, even when the magnetic field is generated by focal sources. Thus, minimum norm estimation and other methods for estimating distributed source models will be less well suited for circumstances where the magnetic field is due to a small number of highly focal sources.

4.2.4 Inverse solutions: spatial filtering

So far, we have looked at methods of solving the inverse problem by fitting the parameters of the source model to the data to find the source configuration that best explains the data. Because sources at each possible location and orientation produce magnetic fields that have a specific spatial pattern across the sensors (as defined by the lead field), an alternative method of estimating the time series of individual sources is to construct a spatial filter that passes that part of the field that follows this spatial pattern, while excluding the parts of the field that are due to other sources or of various noise signals present in the data. This can then be repeated for all possible sources to build an estimate of the source distribution within the head. This method is known as *beamforming*.

The optimal spatial filter for each source location would pass the signal originating from that location while completely removing signals from all other locations. However, because the number of sensors is much fewer than the number of possible sources, it is not possible to create an independent filter for every source location. Instead, the best that can be achieved is to create a spatial filter that minimises the contribution of signals from other locations, rather than removing them completely. The spatial filters necessary to achieve this minimisation will vary depending on the sources that contribute to the data (as well as the presence of any noise signals that need to be filtered out of the data). Thus, the beamforming technique works by adapting the spatial filters to achieve the optimal filtering based on the signals present in the data (for this reason, beamforming is sometimes described as adaptive spatial filtering because the spatial filters are adapted to the data).

If the sources are uncorrelated in time, it is possible to achieve this minimisation by calculating the spatial filter from the covariance of the data across sensors. This is known as *linearly-constrained minimum variance* (LCMV) beamforming (Van Veen et al., 1997), as the resulting spatial filters minimise the variance of the estimated source time-series, subject to the constraint that filter does not supress any signal originating at the source location. Alternatively, the spatial filter can be applied in the frequency domain by measuring the cross-spectral density (this quantifies the relationship between the magnitudes and phases at a pre-specified frequency of interest between pairs of sensors), rather than the covariance, of the data across sensors. This is known as *dynamical imaging of coherent sources* (DICS) (Gross et al., 2001). Regardless of which method is used, the spatial filter is implemented by assigning a weight between each sensor and each source location, and the time series of source moment at the corresponding location is calculated as the weighted sum of the sensor time series.

Beamformers can be applied in one of two ways. In one approach, sources are defined on a grid of points distributed across the brain volume. The data can then be collapsed across time (for instance by calculating source power within a specific time window or contrasted time windows) and represented and analysed as a 3D volumetric image. Alternatively, if the aim is to measure information about individual sources, spatial filters can be calculated for one or more predefined locations, and the time series of source moment can be estimated for each location. This is known as a *virtual sensor* or *virtual electrode* analysis because the technique simulates the process of measuring from an electrode placed at the source location. The time series can then be analysed using the techniques described in Chapter 3.

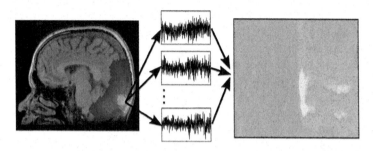

Figure 4.5 Illustration of source analysis using beamforming.

Figure 4.5 illustrates this analysis process. The left panel shows a slice from a beamformer volumetric image displayed on the subject's structural MRI. Virtual sensor time series can then be extracted from a location of interest (here the image location with the largest response) and used as the basis for further analysis such as calculation of the spectrogram of the event-related response.

Beamforming exhibits the reverse depth bias to minimum norm estimation, with sources tending to increase in power as they increase in depth. This is because deeper sources require larger weights to accurately reconstruct the source time series, and this means the contribution of noise signals and signal leakage to the source time series tend to be larger with increasing source depth. It is therefore common to scale the source time series by an estimate of the projected sensor noise to compensate for this.

A key advantage of beamforming is that, because it is not a fitting technique, it does not require the user to make assumptions about the number or spatial distribution of sources to be included in the inverse solution. As beamforming is a spatial filtering approach, it will also tend to filter out noise signals that have a different spatial distribution across the sensors to the brain signals. This means beamformer source estimation is robust to the presence of artefacts in the data (in contrast to fitting approaches which tend to require artefacts to be removed from the data prior to source estimation).

However, beamforming also has disadvantages. The spatial filters are calculated under the assumption that sources are uncorrelated in time and thus beamforming produces inaccuracies when this assumption is not true (although the technique can be robust to moderate levels of correlation between sources; Hadjipapas, Hillebrand, Holliday, Singh, & Barnes, 2005; Van Veen et al., 1997). Because the spatial filters do not eliminate – but only minimise – the contribution of other signals, the estimated time series for each source will contain not just signals from that location but also some leakage from other locations with similar lead fields. This means that beamformer source estimation is also subject to the same problem of signal leakage described for minimum norm estimation.

A further limitation on beamforming is that accurate calculation of the spatial filters depends on accurately estimating the data covariance. This estimate improves as the number of time samples used to measure the data covariance increases. It is recommended that the covariance should be calculated from several times as many time samples as there are sensors (Van Veen et al., 1997), and if signals have been removed from the data in preprocessing (for instance due to temporal filtering or artefact rejection) then the number of samples required may be much larger than this. This means that beamforming is better suited to brain signals that are sustained over an extended period of time and is less well suited to short-duration responses, such as event-related fields.

4.2.5 Summary

In this section we have seen that MEG data can be analysed based on an estimate of the distribution of the underlying source currents. This corresponds to analysing data in source space.

Analysing the data in source space offers the potential for more precise spatial information about the sources of brain responses than can be achieved in sensor space. However, because MEG source estimation is an ill-posed inverse problem, there is no unique set of sources that explain any measured magnetic field. Methods such as model fitting and spatial filtering can be used to constrain the source estimation to a unique solution. These methods create source space representations of the data that can be used for imaging analysis or to extract source time series, but the results are only accurate to the extent that the assumptions underlying the methods holds true for the data.

4.3 Statistical analysis of MEG data

So far, we have looked at the different ways that spatial and temporal aspects of the MEG data can be measured and quantified. However, in most cases MEG data analysis is aimed not just at measuring brain signals but at performing statistical inferences on those measurements, for instance by performing hypothesis testing on the data. Thus, in this final section of the chapter we look at some of the methods that can be used to perform statistical analysis of MEG data.

4.3.1 Statistical inference from MEG data

As we have seen, MEG data is generally too noisy for meaningful information to be extracted from a single set of observations (e.g. from the data sampled within a single epoch). Instead, conditions are usually repeated across multiple epochs (typically corresponding to a series of trials or blocks) to produce repeated measurements for each condition. Once data has been acquired from an individual subject, each data sample (or group of samples) can then be summarised across epochs within each condition for analysis by one or more measures that can be used for statistical inference. This is known as *subject-level* or *first-level* statistical analysis. These can be simple descriptive measures (such as the mean), test statistics (such as the *t*-statistic), or parameters generated by fitting a statistical model to the data (such as the general linear model). These may often be based on contrasts between different time periods within a condition (such as between a period containing an event-related response and a preceding baseline period) or between different conditions.

Usually, the aim is to make statistical inferences about populations rather than individual subjects: either about differences between groups (between-subjects effects) or about differences between conditions within a group (within-subjects effects) or a combination of both. In these cases, data collection involves acquiring data from multiple subjects and performing *group-level* – also known as *second-level* – analysis by collapsing subject-level measures across subjects to produce group-level measures.

Usually, the purpose of generating subject- or group-level measures is to make inferences about experimental hypotheses. This generally involves performing a statistical test to generate a p-value that quantifies the probability of observing the corresponding test statistic under the null hypothesis. If the p-value is found to be below a pre-determined threshold (known as the *significance level*) then the null hypothesis can be rejected, and the results are regarded as statistically significant.

Statistical testing can be performed using parametric tests, such as student's *t*-test or ANOVA, in which the data is assumed to be drawn from a known distribution (typically the normal distribution). However, for many MEG measures the data may not follow a known parametric distribution, and so non-parametric tests are often used instead. By far the most common approach to non-parametric statistic testing used with MEG is permutation testing (Singh et al., 2003). This involves permuting condition labels across trials (for subject-level analysis) or across subjects (for group-level analysis) and recalculating the test statistic for each permutation of the data in order to measure the distribution of the statistic across permutations. The test statistic from the original, unpermuted data can then be compared with this distribution in order to calculate the probability of finding a test statistic more extreme than the observed statistic, and this probability can be compared to the statistical threshold in order to determine whether the null hypothesis of no difference between conditions can be rejected.

Because rejection of the null hypothesis is an inherently probabilistic decision, the process is subject to errors. *Type I errors* (also known as *false positives*) occur when the null hypothesis is rejected despite being true. The rate of type I errors is controlled by the statistical threshold used to reject the null hypothesis (thus, if the threshold for rejection of the null hypothesis is 0.05, then the rate of type I error for each statistical test will be 5%). *Type II errors* (also known as *false negatives*) occur when the null hypothesis is not rejected despite being false. The type II error rate therefore determines the power of the test to detect true experimental effects (this is often known as the *statistical power* of the test). The type II error rate decreases as the size of the experimental effect, the sample size or the statistical threshold increases. The means that, for a given effect and sample size, the rate of type I and II errors are determined by the statistical threshold in opposite directions: as the threshold becomes stricter, type I errors decrease but type II errors increase.

4.3.2 Mass univariate analysis

When analysing MEG data an intuitive approach is to treat each sample in (sensor or source) space and time (and/or frequency) within an epoch as a separate variable. In this case the data at each sample is said to be *univariate* because it represents samples from a single variable. Univariate statistical tests can in theory be performed at a specific sample of interest, but it is rare in practice for a hypothesis to relate to the signal measured at an individual sample. Instead, statistical testing is usually performed on all samples within the data set (or a preselected subset of samples) to test for the presence of experimental effects at any individual sample. This is known as *mass univariate* analysis, because the data is treated as containing a large number (hence mass) of univariate variables (Groppe et al., 2011).

Depending on the number of samples present in the data (which here includes not only samples across time and/or frequency but also across sensors or sources), the mass univariate analysis might require anywhere from thousands to millions of tests to be performed. This leads to what is known as the multiple comparisons problem: as the number of tests increases, the probability of a type I error occurring for any of the tests – known as the *familywise error rate* (FWER) – must also increase. Thus, the chance of finding a significant effect present somewhere in the data when no genuine effect exists anywhere in the data will be much larger than expected from the nominal false positive rate set by the statistical threshold. To maintain accurate control of the type I error rate across the family of tests, it is therefore necessary to reduce the statistical threshold used for the individual tests to compensate for the presence of multiple comparisons (for instance by reducing the threshold in proportion to the number of comparisons – an adjustment known as Bonferroni correction). However, this necessarily reduces the power of the tests to detect genuine effects and therefore increases the number of type II errors. For this reason, an important element of mass univariate testing of MEG data involves adopting approaches to correcting for multiple comparisons that minimise the loss of statistical power.

One approach is to opt to control for a less stringent measure of type I error than the familywise error rate, known as the *false discovery rate* (FDR). This is defined as the expected rate of type I errors across the family of tests. This provides less strict control of the number of false positives, as it controls for the total expected number of type I errors across tests, rather than for the rate that a type I error across any of the tests, but therefore leads to a lower type II error rate. Correction for the false discovery rate is most commonly implemented using a method known as the Benjamini-Hochberg procedure (Benjamini & Hochberg, 1995; Genovese et al., 2002).

Where instead it is considered desirable to control for the familywise error rate, a common approach to correcting for multiple comparisons is to compare the individual test statistics against the null distribution of the maximum test statistic across tests. While it is perhaps not intuitive that it should be the case, comparing against the null distribution of the maximum test statistic across tests ensures accurate control of the familywise error rate but will generally produce fewer type II errors than alternative methods (such as Bonferroni correction). For parametric tests, the null distribution of the maximum can be calculated using methods from a branch of statistics called *random field theory* (Kiebel et al., 1999). However, because MEG data generally does not conform to parametric assumptions, it is more common to apply this correction when using permutation testing. In this case the null distribution of the maximum can be measured by recording the distribution of maximum test statistic across permutations (Nichols & Holmes, 2001).

Mass univariate analysis and correction for multiple comparisons are illustrated in Figure 4.6. The figure shows the group average time series (taken from Perry & Singh, 2014) from a single source for two conditions corresponding to presentation of a face or a matched

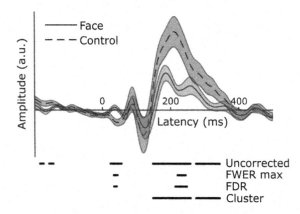

Figure 4.6 Group mean (± standard error) event-related responses to faces and matched control stimuli. The black dashes show statistically significant samples for different forms of correction for multiple comparisons.

control stimulus respectively. The black lines below the plot show the samples in which a significant difference was found to be present (at $p < 0.05$) for different levels of correction for multiple comparisons (as well as for cluster-based analysis which we will look at in the next section). The top row shows the samples found to be significant when no correction is applied. When compared to other rows, it can be seen that this leads to more samples found to have a significant difference, but the lack of correction means that the probability of finding a significant difference anywhere in the data when no genuine effect is present is greater than the nominal false positive rate of 5%. In this example, some significant differences are found prior to stimulus onset (0 seconds), which almost certainly correspond to false positives, as we would not expect differences between conditions prior to stimulus onset.

The second row shows the samples found to be significant when the familywise error rate was controlled at 0.05 (using comparison to the null distribution of the maximum test statistic). We can see that, because this is a more conservative statistical threshold, fewer samples are now significant (compared to the uncorrected test) but with the advantage that the false positive rate across the family of tests is now accurately controlled. The third row shows the samples that were found to be significant when corrections for multiple comparisons was performed by controlling the false discovery rate. Because this is a more liberal correction than controlling for the familywise error rate, we can see that more samples exhibit significant differences than for the second row, but this comes at the cost of less strict control of the false positive rate.

In addition to the methods outlined so far, the effect of the multiple comparisons problem can also be reduced simply by reducing the number of comparisons to be performed. In fMRI, one popular approach has been to adopt a *region of interest* (ROI) approach, in which statistical tests are only performed on voxels within predetermined spatial regions of interest. A similar approach can be applied to MEG by analysing data at pre-selected sensors or sources of interest and/or pre-selected time windows or frequency bands of interest. Because statistical tests are only performed on a subset of samples, this can dramatically reduce the number of comparisons that must be corrected for. This approach is used for the analysis shown in Figure 4.6, where only data from a single source is analysed and only samples for a time window around stimulus onset rather than the full length of the epoch.

The number of comparisons can be reduced even further if, rather than treating each individual sample within a region (or time window or frequency band) of interest as a univariate measure, data is collapsed across samples to produce one or more summary measures (such as the mean or maximum across samples). Statistical testing can then be applied to the summary measures, rather than to the individual samples. We have already encountered an example of this approach when looking at the analysis of event-related responses, where it is common to characterise each component of the response by a single summary measure such as amplitude or latency.

Note however, that to avoid biasing the statistical tests, the criteria used for selecting the samples to analyse (or which summary measures to use) must be independent of the experimental effect itself. For instance, when testing for a difference between conditions, it would not be legitimate to define a region of interest based on those samples that show the largest difference between conditions as this would bias the subsequent tests in favour of rejecting the null hypothesis.

4.3.3 Cluster-based analysis

Mass univariate analysis treats each sample as an independent variable but, because MEG data is locally correlated, this is rarely true in practice. Thus, the problem of multiple comparisons can be reduced (or avoided all together) if approaches to statistical testing are used that look for effects occurring over clusters of samples, rather than treating each sample separately (Maris & Oostenveld, 2007). This is known as *cluster-based analysis*.

Cluster-based analysis is performed by first performing statistical comparisons for individual data samples, as would be performed for a mass univariate analysis. However, rather than using the statistical comparisons to test the null hypothesis, the results of these first-stage comparisons are used to find clusters of samples that exceed the statistical threshold. Each cluster present in the data is then quantified by a cluster-level statistic such as the sum of the test statistic across samples within the cluster (sometimes called the *cluster mass*). Statistical testing is then performed on these cluster-level statistics by calculating the probability that a cluster statistic of equal or greater magnitude would be found anywhere in the data under the null hypothesis.

Under parametric assumptions, the null distribution of the cluster statistics can be calculated using random field theory, but when analysing MEG data, it is more common to calculate the distribution non-parametrically using a permutation test. This calculation is performed by permuting condition labels across subjects (or across conditions for within-subject designs) and repeating the clustering procedure for the permuted data. The cluster statistic is measured for each cluster, the maximum cluster statistic is recorded for each permutation and the distribution of the maximum across permutations forms the null distribution against which the clusters are compared in order to calculate the corresponding p-value. Thus, rather than performing statistical inference on the individual samples, hypothesis testing is performed on the properties of clusters of samples.

To illustrate this procedure, cluster-based analysis was applied to the data shown in Figure 4.6. Data was first thresholded using the uncorrected statistical comparison shown in the 'Uncorrected' row of the figure. These samples formed five clusters of neighbouring samples, shown by the five contiguous lines in the 'Uncorrected' row. The mass of each cluster was calculated, and permutation testing was used to determine the probability of finding a cluster with equal or greater mass under the null hypothesis of no difference between conditions. The two clusters shown on the bottom row (labelled 'Cluster') were found to be significant at $p < 0.05$.

The advantage of cluster-based statistical testing is that experimental effects are tested collectively across clusters meaning that correction for multiple comparisons is unnecessary. However, the disadvantage of this approach is that statistical inferences are only made about properties of the clusters, and not about individual samples. Thus, in the example shown in Figure 3.18, it is not possible to determine if any individual sample shows significant differences between conditions, only that the two significant clusters have greater mass than would be expected by chance. Therefore, while it is possible to determine that differences between conditions exists, it is impossible to localise these differences to precise sensors or sources or to specific latencies or frequencies within the data (see Sassenhagen & Draschkow (2019) for a more detailed discussion of this issue).

4.3.4 Summary

MEG data can be analysed at one of two levels: in first-level analysis statistics are calculated based on repeated measurements (e.g. across epochs) from the individual subject, while second-level analysis involves calculating statistics from first-level measures across subjects. Statistical inference can then be performed by performing hypothesis testing on the first- or second-level statistics. This can take the form of mass univariate analysis, where statistical testing is applied separately for each data sample. However, because this often involves a large number of simultaneous statistical tests, some form of correction for multiple comparisons must be performed in order to maintain an accurate rate of type II (false positive) errors. A commonly used alternative approach to statistical analysis of MEG data that avoids the problem of multiple comparisons is to perform cluster-based analyses. This involves performing statistical tests on clusters of samples containing a common experimental effect of interest, rather than on individual samples.

Further reading

Baillet, S., Mosher J. C., & Leahy, R.M. (2001). Electromagnetic brain mapping, *IEEE Signal Processing Magazine, 18*(6), 14–30. https://doi.org/10.1109/79.962275

Groppe, D. M., Urbach, T. P., & Kutas, M. (2011). Mass univariate analysis of event-related brain potentials/fields I: A critical tutorial review. *Psychophysiology, 48*(12), 1711. https://doi.org/10.1111/J.1469-8986.2011.01273.X

Hämäläinen, M. S., Lin, F-H., & Mosher, J. C. (2010). Anatomically and functionally constrained minimum–norm estimates. In P. C. Hansen, M. L. Kringelbach, & R. Salmelin (Eds.), *MEG: An Introduction to Methods*, 186–215. Oxford University Press. https://doi.org/10.1093/acprof:oso/9780195307238.003.0008

Hillebrand, A. & Barnes, G. R. (2005). Beamformer analysis of MEG data, *International Review of Neurobiology, 68*, 149–171. https://doi.org/10.1016/S0074-7742(05)68006-3

Maris, E. (2012). Statistical testing in electrophysiological studies. *Psychophysiology, 49*(4), 549–65. https://doi.org/10.1111/j.1469-8986.2011.01320.x

Salmelin, R. (2010). Multi-dipole modeling in MEG. In P. C. Hansen, M. L. Kringelbach, & R. Salmelin (Eds.), *MEG: An Introduction to Methods*, 124–155. Oxford University Press. https://doi.org/10.1093/acprof:oso/9780195307238.003.0006

References

Benjamini, Y., & Hochberg, Y. (1995). Controlling the false discovery rate: A practical and powerful approach to multiple testing. *Journal of the Royal Statistical Society: Series B (Methodological), 57*(1). https://doi.org/10.1111/j.2517-6161.1995.tb02031.x

Dale, A. M., Liu, A. K., Fischl, B. R., Buckner, R. L., Belliveau, J. W., Lewine, J. D., & Halgren, E. (2000). Dynamic statistical parametric mapping: Combining fMRI and MEG for high-resolution imaging of cortical activity. *Neuron, 26*(1). https://doi.org/10.1016/S0896-6273(00)81138-1

Fuchs, M., Kastner, J., Wagner, M., Hawes, S., & Ebersole, J. S. (2002). A standardized boundary element method volume conductor model. *Clinical Neurophysiology, 113*(5), 702–712. https://doi.org/10.1016/S1388-2457(02)00030-5

Genovese, C. R., Lazar, N. A., & Nichols, T. (2002). Thresholding of statistical maps in functional neuroimaging using the false discovery rate. *NeuroImage, 15*(4), 870–878. https://doi.org/10.1006/nimg.2001.1037

Groppe, D. M., Urbach, T. P., & Kutas, M. (2011). Mass univariate analysis of event-related brain potentials/fields I: A critical tutorial review. *Psychophysiology, 48*(12), 1711. https://doi.org/10.1111/J.1469-8986.2011.01273.X

Gross, J., Kujala, J., Hämäläinen, M., Timmermann, L., Schnitzler, A., & Salmelin, R. (2001). Dynamic imaging of coherent sources: Studying neural interactions in the human brain. *Proceedings of the National Academy of Sciences of the United States of America, 98*(2). https://doi.org/10.1073/pnas.98.2.694

Hadjipapas, A., Hillebrand, A., Holliday, I. E., Singh, K. D., & Barnes, G. R. (2005). Assessing interactions of linear and nonlinear neuronal sources using MEG beamformers: a proof of concept. *Clinical Neurophysiology, 116*(6), 1300–1313. https://doi.org/10.1016/J.CLINPH.2005.01.014

Hämäläinen, M. S., & Ilmoniemi, R. J. (1994). Interpreting magnetic fields of the brain: minimum norm estimates. *Medical & Biological Engineering & Computing, 32*(1), 35–42. https://doi.org/10.1007/BF02512476

Huang, M. X., Mosher, J. C., & Leahy, R. M. (1999). A sensor-weighted overlapping-sphere head model and exhaustive head model comparison for MEG. *Physics in Medicine and Biology, 44*, 423–440. https://doi.org/10.1088/0031-9155/44/2/010

Jeffs, B., Leahy, R., & Singh, M. (1987). An evaluation of methods for neuromagnetic image reconstruction. *IEEE Transactions on Biomedical Engineering, 34*(9), 713–723. https://doi.org/10.1109/TBME.1987.325996

Kiebel, S. J., Poline, J. B., Friston, K. J., Holmes, A. P., & Worsley, K. J. (1999). Robust smoothness estimation in statistical parametric maps using standardized residuals from the general linear model. *NeuroImage, 10*(6), 756–766. https://doi.org/10.1006/NIMG.1999.0508

Maris, E., & Oostenveld, R. (2007). Nonparametric statistical testing of EEG- and MEG-data. *Journal of Neuroscience Methods*, *164*(1), 177–190. https://doi.org/10.1016/j.jneumeth.2007.03.024

Mosher, J. C., Lewis, P. S., & Leahy, R. M. (1992). Multiple dipole modeling and localization from spatio-temporal MEG data. *IEEE Transactions on Biomedical Engineering*, *39*(6), 541–557. https://doi.org/10.1109/10.141192

Nichols, T. E., & Holmes, A. P. (2001). Nonparametric permutation tests for functional neuroimaging: a primer with examples. *Human Brain Mapping*, *15*, 1–25. http://onlinelibrary.wiley.com/doi/10.1002/hbm.1058/full

Nolte, G. (2003). The magnetic lead field theorem in the quasi-static approximation and its use for magnetoenchephalography forward calculation in realistic volume conductors. *Physics in Medicine and Biology*, *48*(22). https://doi.org/10.1088/0031-9155/48/22/002

Oostendorp, T. F., & Van Oosterom, A. (1989). Source parameter estimation in inhomogeneous volume conductors of arbitrary shape. *IEEE Transactions on Biomedical Engineering*, *36*(3). https://doi.org/10.1109/10.19859

Pascual-Marqui, R. D. (2002). Standardized low-resolution brain electromagnetic tomography (sLORETA): Technical details. *Methods and Findings in Experimental and Clinical Pharmacology*, *24*(SUPPL. D).

Perry, G., & Singh, K. D. (2014). Localizing evoked and induced responses to faces using magnetoencephalography. *European Journal of Neuroscience*, *39*(October 2013), 1517–1527. https://doi.org/10.1111/ejn.12520

Sassenhagen, J., & Draschkow, D. (2019). Cluster-based permutation tests of MEG/EEG data do not establish significance of effect latency or location. *Psychophysiology*, *56*(6), e13335. https://doi.org/10.1111/PSYP.13335

Sarvas, J. (1987). Basic mathematical and electromagnetic concepts of the biomagnetic inverse problem. *Physics in Medicine and Biology*, *32*(1), 11–22. https://doi.org/10.1088/0031-9155/32/1/004

Singh, K. D., Barnes, G. R., & Hillebrand, A. (2003). Group imaging of task-related changes in cortical synchronisation using nonparametric permutation testing. *NeuroImage*, *19*(4), 1589–1601. https://doi.org/10.1016/S1053-8119(03)00249-0

Van Veen, B. D., Van Drongelen, W., Yuchtman, M., & Suzuki, A. (1997). Localization of brain electrical activity via linearly constrained minimum variance spatial filtering. *IEEE Transactions on Biomedical Engineering*, *44*(9). https://doi.org/10.1109/10.623056

Vorwerk, J., Cho, J. H., Rampp, S., Hamer, H., Knösche, T. R., & Wolters, C. H. (2014). A guideline for head volume conductor modeling in EEG and MEG. *NeuroImage, 100*, 590–607. https://doi.org/10.1016/J.NEU ROIMAGE.2014.06.040

Wang, L., Jensen, O., Van den Brink, D., Weder, N., Schoffelen, J. M., Magyari, L., Hagoort, P., & Bastiaansen, M. (2012). Beta oscillations relate to the N400m during language comprehension. *Human Brain Mapping, 33*(12). https://doi.org/10.1002/hbm.21410

Chapter 5

Applications of MEG

In the previous two chapters we have looked in an abstract sense at how MEG data analysis is performed. In this concluding chapter, we will look at some of the applications of MEG in both research and clinic in order to illustrate how these data analysis techniques are applied in practice.

MEG has a broad range of applications, but in research settings MEG has most frequently been used to measure event-related responses. Thus, in the first section of the chapter we will look at the kinds of event-related responses that can be measured with MEG and present some illustrative examples of how event-related responses have been measured in a selection of research studies. In recent years, a second research application of MEG that has grown in use is the measurement of brain connectivity, and thus in the second section we explore how MEG can be used for this application. Finally, in addition to its research applications, MEG also has applications in medicine. Currently the most widely used clinical application of MEG is in the pre-surgical evaluation of epilepsy patients. Thus, we will conclude the chapter by exploring how MEG is used in clinic for this purpose.

5.1 Event-related responses

Throughout the history of MEG, its most frequent use has been the measurement of event-related responses linked to the perceptual, cognitive and motor processes of the brain. As described in previous chapters, these are brain responses which are time-locked to an

DOI: 10.4324/9781315205175-7

experimental event of interest (such as the presentation of a sensory stimulus or the initiation of a behavioural response). The strength of MEG is that it not only allows the measurement of event-related responses with high levels of precision in time or frequency, but also makes it possible to localise the source(s) of those responses using methods for source estimation.

Event-related responses that can be measured with MEG can be grouped into two categories of response: evoked and induced responses. In this section we will look at example studies that illustrate how these two kinds of response may be measured.

5.1.1 Evoked responses

As covered in the previous chapter, responses that are time-locked to an experimental event (and are also phase-locked to the event in the case of periodic responses) can be measured by averaging data in the time domain. Event-related responses that can be measured using time domain averaging are known as *evoked* responses.

The measurement of evoked responses with MEG has been strongly influenced by research conducted in EEG, where the technique of measuring event-related potentials from trial averaged data has a long history. It has therefore been popular to use trial averaging of MEG data to measure the equivalent event-related fields. Different types of experimental event typically trigger a series of these potentials/fields, which reflect transient changes in the source currents underlying the corresponding brain processes. These responses are measured by averaging (and baseline correcting) the data across epochs time-locked to a specific experimental event of interest. Band-pass filtering is also often applied to the data in order to suppress low and high frequency noise signals and make the timecourse of the evoked response clearer, although some argue against this practice on the basis that filtering can alter the timing of the responses within the data (de Cheveigné & Nelken, 2019).

An illustration of both event-related potentials and fields is shown in Figure 5.1, taken from the work of Shahin and colleagues (Shahin et al., 2005). The data shown are group average evoked responses to auditory tones measured simultaneously with

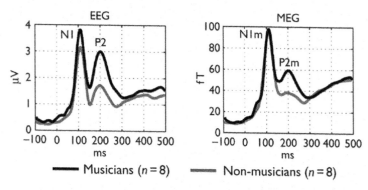

Figure 5.1 Evoked response to an auditory stimulus measured from two groups (musicians and non-musicians) using both EEG and MEG. *Reprinted from Shahin et al. (2005). Modulation of P2 auditory-evoked responses by the spectral complexity of musical sounds. NeuroReport, 16(16), 1781–1785. https://doi.org/10.1097/01.wnr.0000185017.29316.63.*

EEG and MEG from two participant groups (musicians and non-musicians). For simplicity of visualisation, data in these plots has been collapsed across sensors by calculating the root-mean-square amplitude at each time sample, but more typically data would be plotted for individual sensors (or sources). In the event-related potential data, two peaks in the amplitude of the response are present, labelled N1 and P2 respectively (based on whether the potential across the front of the head is negative or positive). Equivalent event-related fields are also present in the MEG data (here labelled by analogy to the EEG data as N1m and P2m), although the EEG and MEG data are not identical (reflecting the fact that the two techniques have different sensitivity to sources within the brain depending on the position and orientation of those sources). Analysis of the data then takes the form of comparing properties of the evoked response (for instance, the amplitude or latency of specific components) either between conditions in within-subject designs or (as in the example shown here) between groups in between-subject designs.

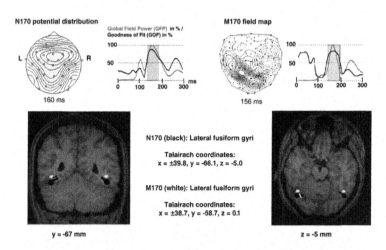

Figure 5.2 EEG and MEG sensor space plots and dipole fits of evoked response to visual presentation of faces. *Reprinted from Neurolmage, 35(4), Deffke et al., MEG/EEG sources of the 170-ms response to faces are co-localized in the fusiform gyrus, 1495–1501, Copyright (2007), with permission from Elsevier.*

Measurement of event-related fields is not restricted to simple stimuli such as auditory tones but can also be applied to the measurement of responses in higher-level sensory areas to complex sensory stimuli. One example of this is the use of MEG to study evoked responses to faces. Figure 5.2 shows the results of one such study in which Deffke and colleagues (Deffke et al., 2007) made simultaneous measurements of EEG and MEG while participants viewed images of faces. The figure shows the potential distribution and magnetic field map of an event-related response occurring around 170 ms (known as the N170 event-related potential and the M170 event-related field) that is known to be elicited more strongly to faces than to other categories of visual stimuli. Measurement of evoked responses is not restricted to sensor space but can also be performed in source space. In this study they used dipole fitting to estimate the source of the MEG (black circles) and EEG (white circles) evoked responses. The results show consistent source localisation between the two modalities to a location in the brain (the fusiform gyrus) that is known to be involved in face processing (Kanwisher & Yovel, 2006).

In many cases it may not be possible to assume that evoked responses are generated by a small number of focal sources, and therefore it is more common to use either distributed source models or beamforming to measure evoked responses in source space. An example of this is shown in Figure 5.3 taken from a study by Halgren and colleagues (Halgren et al., 2002) in which they presented subjects with sentences containing either semantically congruent or

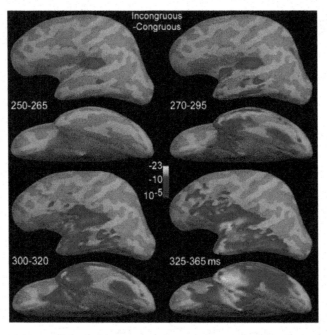

Figure 5.3 Cortical surface maps of the statistical difference in source power between congruous and incongruous sentence endings during four time intervals. *Reprinted from NeuroImage, 17(3), Halgren et al., N400-like magnetoencephalography responses modulated by semantic context, word frequency and lexical class in sentences, 1101–1116, Copyright (2002), with permission from Elsevier.*

incongruent endings. For the results shown, they used dynamical statistical parametric mapping – a variant of minimum norm estimation – to estimate the source distribution across the cortical surface, creating two-dimensional surface maps of source currents for each condition. They then performed a mass univariate analysis of the difference between the congruent and incongruent conditions for mean source power within several time windows in order to map differences in source activity between conditions over time. Figure 5.3 shows maps of p-values measured from the statistical contrast between conditions for each time window. The contrasts show enhanced source activity for incongruous relative to congruous sentence endings in the left hemisphere, beginning in Wernicke's area around 250 ms and subsequently spreading to the anterior temporal lobe and frontal cortex. Thus, the figure illustrates how distributed source models can be used to localise evoked responses that are generated by a distributed pattern of sources, and how the resulting source solutions can be analysed as surface maps of source power.

5.1.2 Induced responses

Awareness that electrophysiological signals contain identifiable rhythms dates back to the first EEG recordings, made by the German psychiatrist Hans Berger in the 1920s (Berger, 1929). Berger observed that recordings made with EEG contained two spontaneously occurring rhythms when subjects were at a state of rest, one with a frequency around 10 Hz that he named the alpha wave and the second with a frequency around 25 Hz that he named the beta wave. The work of subsequent researchers led to the discovery of other state-dependent rhythms of the EEG and to the loose categorisation of those signals based on their frequency: delta (1–4 Hz), theta (4–7 Hz), alpha (8–15 Hz), beta (15–30 Hz) & gamma (>30 Hz).

These rhythms can exhibit event-related increases and decreases in power (the latter case can occur when spontaneous rhythms present in the baseline time interval decrease in power during sensory stimulation or task performance) and therefore represent a second kind of event-related response that can be measured using MEG. These are known as *induced* responses. Because these power changes are thought to reflect changes in rhythmical currents that are synchronous across neurons, event-related increases and decreases in power are sometimes also referred to as *event-related synchronisation* (ERS) and *event-related desynchronization* (ERD) respectively.

In some cases, these rhythms may have a consistent phase across epochs (i.e. they are phase-locked to the experimental event), and therefore can be measured after averaging data in the time domain and treated as a type of evoked response. More commonly, the phase of the rhythm varies between epochs and the response therefore tends to average out of the time-domain average. Instead, event-related changes in these rhythms must be measured in the frequency and time–frequency domain. Changes in these non-phase-locked rhythms constitute the induced response.

One example of an event-related response that contains both increases and decreases of power is the induced response generated in sensorimotor cortex related to voluntary initiation of a movement. Figure 5.4 shows an example of this response taken from a study by Jurkiewicz and colleagues (Jurkiewicz et al., 2006) in which MEG was measured while subjects performed abductions of their right-hand index finger. The figure shows group average spectrograms

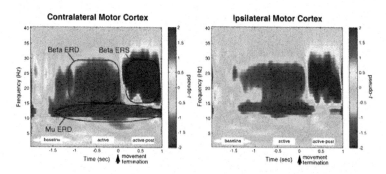

Figure 5.4 Spectrograms of the induced response to abduction of the right index finger, measured from the motor cortices contralateral and ipsilateral to the right hand. *Reprinted from NeuroImage, 32(3), Jurkiewicz et al., Post-movement beta rebound is generated in motor cortex: Evidence from neuromagnetic recordings, 1281–1289, Copyright (2006), with permission from Elsevier.*

of virtual sensors (measured using beamforming) from sources in the region of contralateral (left) and ipsilateral (right) central sulcus containing the representation of the hand. Data epochs were time-locked to movement termination to measure event-related responses linked to finger movement.

In the beta frequency range, an event-related decrease of power occurs before movement termination (that is, occurring prior to and during the movement), reflecting a suppression of the spontaneous beta rhythm. This is followed by an increase of power after the movement terminates. Additionally, a sustained power decrease in the alpha frequency band (this corresponds to the suppression of a rhythm occurring in the motor cortex known as the mu rhythm) during a time interval overlapping with that of the beta power changes. This shows that induced responses can occur at multiple frequency bands and time intervals and may correspond to increases or decreases in power (or a combination of both).

As with evoked responses, within-subjects or between-subjects comparisons can be performed between induced responses to look for experimental differences between conditions or groups. One example of this is shown in Figure 5.5, taken from research conducted by Hamandi and colleagues (Hamandi et al., 2011) into

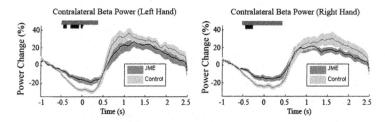

Figure 5.5 Power envelopes of the beta response to abduction of the left or right index fingers for patients with juvenile myoclonic epilepsy (JME) and non-epileptic controls, measured from the contralateral motor cortex. *Reprinted from Clinical Neurophysiology, 122(11), Hamandi, Singh & Muthukumaraswamy, Reduced movement-related beta desynchronisation in juvenile myoclonic epilepsy: A MEG study of task specific cortical modulation, 2128–2138, Copyright (2011), with permission from the International Federation of Clinical Neurophysiology.*

juvenile myoclonic epilepsy (JME). This is a form of epilepsy that is first seen in childhood and is characterised by frequent involuntary jerks in the arms or legs. To investigate whether these involuntary movements might reflect alterations in motor cortex functions in these patients, Hamandi and colleagues compared the induced response to finger abduction between a group of patients with this form of epilepsy and a group of non-epileptic control subjects.

As in the previous study, beamforming was used to estimate virtual sensor time series from sources in the area around the central sulcus corresponding to the representation of the hand (data is plotted here for the contralateral cortex only). Figure 5.5 shows the envelope of power (i.e. the time series of instantaneous power) in the beta frequency range for each of the two groups and for movements made with each hand. The black and grey bars above the plots indicate samples in which the power envelope was significantly different between groups both with (black) and without (grey) correction for multiple comparisons. Differences in the event-related responses at this frequency can be seen between the two groups, but these differences are only significant for the decrease in beta power prior to movement onset and not for the increase in beta power following movement termination. This shows that experimental differences in the induced response may occur for one component of the response but not for others, illustrating why it is often necessary to identify and analyse the different components of the response.

Another example of an induced response that has been heavily studied with MEG (and EEG) is the modulation of the spontaneous alpha rhythm in sensory cortices by attentional cues. For instance, where individuals are cued to attend to their left or right side, a corresponding lateralisation of the alpha rhythm is seen: power decreases in the hemisphere that processes information from the attended side of the visual field and increases in power in the opposite hemisphere.

One example of this shown in Figure 5.6, taken from the work of Haegens and colleagues (Haegens et al., 2011). The data shown is taken from a somatosensory attention task in which participants were visually cued to attend to the right or left hand prior to performing discrimination of a somatosensory stimulus presented to the attended

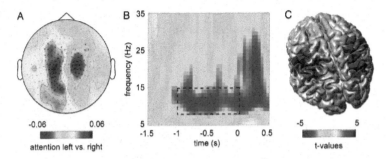

Figure 5.6 (A) Sensor space contrast of alpha power in response to the cueing of attention to the left vs right hand. (B) Spectrogram of alpha power decrease in response to the attentional cue. (C) Source space estimation of contrast shown in A. *Reprinted from Haegens, Händel & Jensen (2011), with permission from the Society for Neuroscience.*

hand. Figure 5.6 A shows difference in alpha power for left versus right attention measured in sensor space using a planar gradient representation of the data. The figure reveals that lateralisation of attention leads to a difference in the lateralisation of alpha power over central sensors. A spectrogram of the alpha power decrease following the cue (Figure 5.6 B) shows that this effect emerges prior to the onset (corresponding to 0 seconds on the time axis) of the stimulus used in the discrimination task, meaning that the lateralisation in alpha power was a response to the visual cue rather than to the somatosensory stimulus.

Source maps produced using beamforming demonstrate that the alpha lateralisation is localised to bilateral regions of the parietal cortex involved in somatosensory processing (Figure 5.6 C). This illustrates how information about the timing and localisation of event-related responses can be used to identify the functional role of those responses: the change in lateralisation of alpha power occurs at the time of the visual cue, but because it occurs in areas of cortex involved in somatosensory processing, it is unlikely to reflect sensory processing of the cue but is instead likely to reflect a shift in attention to somatosensory representation of the cued hand. In support of this,

Haegens and colleagues found that the level of alpha lateralisation decreased as the visual cue became less reliable in signalling the side that the somatosensory stimulus would be presented, and that greater levels of alpha lateralisation corresponded to greater performance on the discrimination task.

5.1.3 Summary

A major application of MEG is the measurement of event-related brain responses. These can be categorised into two types of response. Evoked responses are time-locked to an experimental event and can be analysed by averaging data across epochs in the time domain. Induced responses are event-related power changes in brain rhythms that are not phase-locked to the experimental event and therefore must be analysed by averaging data in the frequency or time-frequency domains.

Evoked responses typically correspond to a series of transient changes in the magnetic field, known as event-related fields. Measurement of properties of these fields, such as their amplitude or latency, can be used to investigate the underlying perceptual, cognitive and motor processes that generate these fields, while source analysis techniques can be used to estimate the anatomical source of the fields.

Induced responses typically correspond to event-related changes (both decreases and increases) of power within specific frequency bands. As with measurement of evoked responses, measurement of properties of induced responses (in this case parameters such as power, frequency and phase) can be used to investigate a variety of psychological processes.

5.2 Functional connectivity

Brain function is rarely the result of activity within a single brain area but instead is the outcome of coordinated activity within networks of interconnected regions. Therefore, in order to understand brain function it is necessary not only to understand the functional role of individual brain regions, but also how those regions are connected in order to form functional networks. For this reason, measurement of brain connectivity is an application of MEG that has become of increasing importance in recent years.

Where two sources in the brain are connected, this should create some form of statistical relationship between their time series. Therefore, in MEG research, connectivity is quantified by the measurement of statistical relationships in data time series measured from different sensors or sources. This is known as *functional connectivity* (in contrast to *structural connectivity* which is defined as the presence of anatomical connections between areas and is measured using MRI). In this section we will look at the general principles of how functional connectivity is measured from MEG data, as well as examples of how those methods have been applied in practice. Although it is possible to measure functional connectivity while participants perform experimental tasks, it is currently more common to measure connectivity from data collected while participants are at rest. Thus, here we will focus specifically on measurement of resting state functional connectivity.

5.2.1 Measuring functional connectivity

Functional connectivity is defined by the presence of statistical relationships between the time series of sensors or sources. These relationships are usually measured between pairs of time series (known as *bivariate* connectivity), although methods also exist to measure statistical interactions amongst larger numbers of time series (known as *multivariate* connectivity). Pairwise connectivity can be measured between pre-determined pairs of sensors or sources, by designating an individual sensor or source as a 'seed' and measuring its pairwise connectivity with all other sensors or sources, or by measuring connectivity for all pairwise combinations of sensors or sources.

In general, the choice of which pairwise connections to measure represent a trade-off. The more connections that are measured, the greater the extent of connectivity that can be quantified and the lower the likelihood that connectivity may be missed. However, the more connections that are measured the more complicated and time consuming the results are to analyse and interpret and the less statistical power there is to detect differences in those connections between groups due to the need to correct for multiple comparisons. This is a particular problem when working in source space, where the source estimate may contain many thousands of sources, leading to a combinatorial explosion of possible pairwise connections amongst sources.

There are many different types of statistical relationship that might exist between data time series, and therefore there are many different methods to quantify functional connectivity. These differ in a variety of respects:

- whether they measure statistical relationships in the time or frequency domain,
- whether they are directed (meaning that the measurement of connectivity from location A → location B may differ from the measurement from location B → location A) or non-directed (meaning that there is only a single measurement of connectivity between each pair of locations),
- whether they assume a linear or non-linear relationship between the time series,
- whether they measure statistical relationships that are instantaneous in time or that occur with a time delay,
- whether they assume that connectivity is stationary (meaning that the connectivity between sensors or sources does not change over the course of the time series) or non-stationary (meaning that connectivity varies over time).

What all these measures have in common is that they measure the presence of a statistical relationship between sensors or sources. However, although the presence of a statistical relationship is often assumed to imply a causal relationship, this is not always the case. For instance, the time series of a pair of sources may be statistically related to each other due to sharing a common input or because they are connected via one or more intermediate sources rather than because they are connected to each other. The presence and strength of noise signals and various data artefacts can also affect the statistical relationship between data time series. Therefore, caution must be taken when interpreting measurements of functional connectivity, and where the aim is to establish causal connection between sources (this is known as *effective connectivity*) then more advanced techniques based on mathematical modelling of the underlying network structure must be used (Kiebel et al., 2008).

In addition, a practical difficulty for the researcher wishing to measure functional connectivity is that there is a proliferation of different measures that can be used to measure connectivity, each based on different assumptions about the type of statistical relationship that indicates the presence of connectivity. These different methods will tend to give different results and it may be difficult to determine which is the most appropriate method to use for a given data set and research question. This also means that it is not possible to give a comprehensive summary of all possible methods here (and indeed any attempt to produce a comprehensive summary is likely to become out of date quickly, as new methods are introduced frequently). Instead, to illustrate how the analysis of connectivity is applied in practice, we will focus here on two of the most widely used methods (for a more extensive list of methods see van Diessen et al., 2015).

5.2.2 Phase coherence

Where two locations in the brain exhibit functional connectivity, one way that this connectivity might be exhibited is through coupling of the phases of the two data time series. Thus, one widely used approach to measuring functional connectivity is to quantify the extent to which measurements of phase (measured from a frequency of interest) show a consistent relationship between sensors or sources.

In Chapter 3 we have seen that the consistency in phase of a signal across epochs can be quantified using a measure known as phase coherence. This can also be used to quantify connectivity if, instead of measuring the consistency of the phase of the data from the time series of a single sensor or source, it is instead used to quantifying the consistency of the *difference* in phase measured between a pair of sensors or sources. This can be measured either across

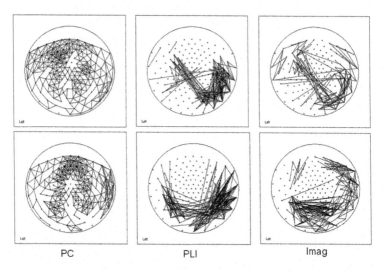

PC   PLI   Imag

Figure 5.7 Maps of sensor pairs showing above threshold connectivity measured in two subjects using phase coherence (PC), the phase lag index (PLI) and the imaginary part of coherence (Imag). *Reprinted from Stam, Nolte & Daffertshofer (2007) Phase lag index: Assessment of functional connectivity from multi channel EEG and MEG with diminished bias from common sources, Human Brain Mapping,* © *2007 Wiley-Liss, Inc.*

epochs or more commonly across time samples (using measures of instantaneous phase). An example of this can be seen in the left panel of Figure 5.7, which shows sensor-level connectivity for two subjects measured from resting data (Stam et al., 2007). The lines connecting sensors show those pairs of sensors with high levels of phase coherence.

The results shown in these two plots show connectivity primarily occurring over short distances (largely between neighbouring sensors). This demonstrates a major methodological issue that effects all attempts to quantify connectivity from MEG data. Because the magnetic field of each source spreads over multiple sensors due to field spread, pairs of sensors may have a statistical relationship between their time series due to measuring the same source, rather than because they are measuring connectivity between two separate sources. A similar effect also occurs in source space, where signal leakage can create a statistical relationship between pairs of sources with similar lead fields. Thus, the presence of field spread (and signal leakage in source space) can introduce spurious connectivity amongst sensors (or sources) that are close together.

The statistical relationships caused by field spread and signal leakage have the property that they must occur instantaneously (i.e. they must occur at the same time sample). These are often known as *zero lag* (or, in the frequency domain, *zero phase lag*) effects, because they occur without any time delay. Therefore, one approach to prevent these effects from influencing connectivity is to only measure statistical relationships that are delayed in time. When measuring connectivity based on phase, this corresponds to measuring the extent to which pairs of sensors or sources have phases that show a consistent, *non-zero* phase difference. The central and right panels of Figure 5.7 shows connectivity measured from the same data but with two alternative phase-based metrics that measure the presence of consistent, non–zero phase difference between pairs of time series: the *imaginary part of coherence* (sometimes known as *imaginary coherence*; Nolte et al., 2004) and the *phase lag index* (Stam et al., 2007).

We can see that when connectivity is measured using either of these alternative methods, the strongest connections are no longer amongst neighbouring sensors, suggesting that the results now reflect genuine connectivity rather than spurious local connectivity due to field spread. Note, however, that the pattern of connectivity although similar, is not identical in the central and right panels. This illustrates the fact that the results of connectivity analysis are sensitive to the specific connectivity measure used.

To illustrate how these methods are used to answer research questions, Figure 5.8 shows measurements of resting state connectivity in source space (measured using beamforming) in both a control group (Figure 5.8 A) and a group of patients with Alzheimer's disease (Figure 5.8 B) made by Engels and colleagues (Engels et al., 2017). To limit the number of possible pairwise connections between

A. HC   B. AD

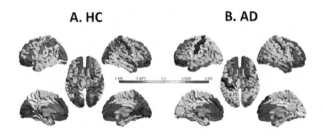

Figure 5.8 Mean directed connectivity measured for 78 anatomical regions of interest in both (A) a healthy control group (HC) and (B) an Alzheimer's disease group (AD). *Reprinted from Neurolmage: Clinical, 15, Engels et al., Directional information flow in patients with Alzheimer's disease. A source-space resting-state MEG study, 673–681, Copyright (2017), with permission from Elsevier.*

sources, they segmented the cortex into 78 regions of interest based on an anatomical atlas and represented each region of interest with a single source time series. This limited the pairwise connections to each of the 78 ROIs (i.e. 78 x 78 connections) rather than between combinations of the many thousands of sources in the original beamformer source estimate of the data.

Pairwise connectivity was measured using *directed phase transfer entropy*, a measure of phase coherence between time series that quantifies the direction (rather than just the strength) of connectivity between two sources. The figure shows the average value of directed connectivity for each of the 78 anatomical regions, where values greater than 0.5 indicate a tendency for connectivity to be directed away from the corresponding region and values below 0.5 indicate a tendency for connectivity to be directed toward the region. The data for the healthy control group shows a pattern of connectivity directed from posterior to anterior regions, but this pattern is not evident in the Alzheimer's group, suggesting that those suffering from disease have altered connectivity compared to the control group. This illustrates one example of the way measures of functional connectivity can be used to identify between-group differences in brain connectivity.

5.2.3 Power envelope correlation

The measurement of resting state connectivity originates in fMRI research where it was first noted by Biswal and colleagues (Biswal et al., 1995) that, when participants are at a rest, low frequency fluctuations in the bold oxygenation level dependent (BOLD) signal are correlated across regions in the brain that are functionally related. Because these correlations cannot be due to task-related changes in the BOLD response, it was inferred that they must instead reflect the presence of functional connectivity between the corresponding brain regions. Thus, measurements of resting fMRI signals have been used to identify functional networks within the brain, and to explore how those networks may be altered in various clinical conditions.

A similar approach to measuring functional connectivity can be applied to MEG resting state data, by measuring low frequency changes in the envelope of the MEG source time series. This approach is illustrated in Figure 5.9a, taken from the work of Hipp and colleagues (Hipp et al., 2012). To measure connectivity between two source locations (indicated by white dots) the source times series are bandpass filtered at a frequency band of interest and the power envelopes (represented by the red and blue lines) are measured from the filtered time series. The statistical relationship between the envelope time series can then be quantified using simple correlational measures. This measure of connectivity is known as *power envelope correlation*.

Figure 5.9b shows the correlation of the 16 Hz envelope between a seed source in motor cortex (indicted by a white dot) and with all other sources in an axial slice of the brain (where source time series were estimated from resting data using beamforming), averaged across 43 subjects. Because connectivity is measured here based on the instantaneous correlation (i.e. with zero time lag between the pairs of time series), the results are dominated by signal leakage, reflected by the fact that the strongest correlations present in Figure 5.9b are for sources closest to the seed location (just as the results shown in the left panel of Figure 5.7 shows connectivity amongst neighbouring sensors due to field spread). Thus, it is generally necessary to perform some form of correction for field spread or signal leakage when measuring connectivity using power envelope correlations.

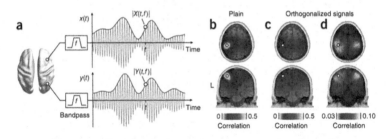

Figure 5.9 (a) Illustration of the measurement of power envelopes from two source locations; (b) Resting state power envelope correlation of each source with a seed location in motor cortex (white circle); (c) The same correlation after orthogonalisation of sources; (d) As c but with the scale adjusted to range between the minimum and maximum correlations. *Reprinted by permission from Springer Nature Customer Service Centre GmbH: Nature, Nature Neuroscience, Large-scale cortical correlation structure of spontaneous oscillatory activity, Hipp et al., Copyright 2012.*

In their study Hipp and colleagues corrected for signal leakage using an orthogonalisation procedure in which each pair of time series was adjusted so that their phases had a difference of ±90°. This abolishes any zero lag correlations between the source time series but not between their power envelopes. Figure 5.9c shows the effects of applying the orthogonalisation: the strong correlation with sources close to the seed is eliminated due to the suppression of signal leakage. When the plot is rescaled (Figure 5.9d) a more distributed pattern of connectivity is apparent, including connectivity with the contralateral motor cortex. This inter-hemispheric connectivity cannot be explained by signal leakage (due to the distance between the sources) and therefore must reflect genuine functional connectivity between the motor cortices during the resting state.

As noted earlier, research into resting connectivity using fMRI has identified the presence of multiple functional networks in the brain. Brookes and colleagues (Brookes et al., 2011) have demonstrated that similar resting state networks can be measured from the power envelopes of MEG source time series. They used the methods described above to measure the source power envelopes, but rather than calculating pairwise correlations between sources, used independent component analysis to separate the data into different spatial networks. The spatial distribution of many of these networks matched those found after applying independent component analysis to fMRI data, indicating that there is some similarity in the patterns of connectivity that can be measured based on MEG power envelopes and those that are measured from the fMRI BOLD signal. Alterations in the structure of these networks have been investigated in a variety of conditions such as Alzheimer's disease (Koelewijn et al., 2017), depression (Nugent et al., 2015) and epilepsy (Koelewijn et al., 2015)

5.2.4 Summary

Brain function is usually not the result of processing in a single brain area but instead the result of processing in networks of brain areas. Thus, the measurement of functional connectivity is an application of MEG that is growing in use. Functional connectivity is quantified by measuring the presence of statistical relationships amongst the sensor or source time series.

There are many types of statistical relationship that might exist between time series, and therefore many different measures of connectivity that are in use. We have looked at two of the most popular approaches here. In the first approach, connectivity is quantified by measuring the consistency of the difference in phase between pairs of sensors or sources. In the second approach, connectivity is quantified by measuring the correlation in the envelope of instantaneous power between pairs of sensors or sources.

An important issue that needs to be dealt with when measuring connectivity from MEG data is that pairs of sensors may show a statistical relationship due to the effects of field spread rather than due to measuring two different, but connected, sources. A similar problem occurs in source space where signal leakage can create statistical relationships among sources even where they are not connected. These effects need to be avoided, either by using measures of connectivity that are insensitive to zero lag connectivity or by transforming the data time series to remove the presence of zero lag correlations.

5.3 Clinical applications of MEG

5.3.1 Pre-surgical evaluation in epilepsy

So far, we have looked at the applications of MEG in research, but MEG can also be used in clinic, particularly in the treatment of epilepsy. To conclude this chapter, we will look briefly at the application of MEG to pre-surgical evaluation in epilepsy.

Epilepsy is a clinical condition characterised by abnormal electrophysiological activity that triggers seizures characterised by temporary loss of awareness, involuntary jerking movements and/or other unusual behaviours and sensations. Epileptic seizures usually do not have any external trigger but instead occur spontaneously (the exception being the class of epilepsy syndromes known as reflex epilepsies in which seizures can be triggered by external stimulation such as flickering light). When EEG is measured during an epileptic seizure a series of rapidly occurring spikes in the electrical potential can usually be observed. These epileptiform spikes may also occur spontaneously between seizures (spikes occurring during seizures are said to be *ictal* and those occurring between seizures are described as *interictal*).

There are many different drug treatments available for epilepsy and patients often become seizure free when treated with one or more of these medications. However, in a minority of cases the epilepsy is drug resistant. In these cases, it is sometimes possible to identify a discrete area of the cortex that acts as the source of the epileptic activity (this is known as the *epileptogenic zone*) and to eliminate the seizures (or at least reduce their frequency) by surgically resecting that area. In order to perform this surgery it is therefore necessary to identify if a clear epileptogenic zone exists and, if so, where in the brain it is located.

Several sources of evidence can be used to identify the epileptogenic zone. In some cases, epilepsy may be caused by the presence of a brain lesion or structural abnormality whose location can be visually identified from the patient's MRI. Alternatively, the epileptogenic zone may be identified by localised changes in metabolism measured using fMRI, PET or SPECT. However, structural and metabolic abnormalities may be incidental findings unrelated to the patient's epilepsy, meaning that these methods cannot be treated as definitively localising the epileptogenic zone.

More direct evidence for the location of the epileptogenic zone can be provided by localising the origin of the epileptiform spikes. As noted, these can be measured using scalp EEG, but the low spatial resolution of EEG and the difficulty of accurately localising the source of the spiking activity (due to the dependency of the measurements on the conductive properties of the various tissues that lay between the source and the scalp) make it poorly suited for this purpose. This has led to clinicians using intracranial EEG recordings (also known as *electrocorticography*) as an alternative means to accurately localise the source(s) of epileptiform spikes. These recordings are made by temporarily removing a section of the patient's skull (a surgical procedure known as a *craniotomy*) and placing a grid of electrodes across the outer surface of the cortex. Alternatively, if the source of epileptiform spikes is thought to originate in a deep brain structure such as the hippocampus, depth electrodes are inserted into the brain tissue.

Because the spatial distribution of the volume current is mainly distorted by the skull (which has a low conductivity), placing the electrodes directly on or in the brain allows for more accurate source localisation than with electrodes placed on the scalp. However, the fact that this technique involves an invasive surgical procedure means that it requires a period of hospital admission for the patient and runs the risk of medical complications. The electrodes also do not provide whole head coverage but instead measure only from the part of the brain exposed by the craniotomy, meaning that some prior estimate of the location of the epileptogenic zone is needed to guide their placement.

Because epileptiform spikes can often be measured by MEG and because the technique is non-invasive, can be performed in a single outpatient visit and provides whole head coverage, many epilepsy clinics have begun exploring the use of MEG as a method for identifying the epileptogenic zone. If the source of epileptiform spikes can be identified with MEG, this can then be used both as an estimate of the location of the epileptogenic zone and as a means to guide the placement of intracranial electrodes for confirmation of that estimate.

A typical MEG protocol for spike localisation involves one or more data acquisitions while the patient is at rest, in order to measure spontaneously occurring epileptiform spikes. As it is necessary for participants to remain still (to prevent the MEG data from being affected by head movements) this generally involves measurements of interictal spikes although some clinics have experimented with measuring epileptiform spikes occurring during seizures (for a review of this topic, see Stefan & Rampp, 2020). Because spiking activity is spontaneous, the timing of the response cannot be linked to an external event. For this reason, it is necessary to perform post-hoc identification of the timing of each spike within the data in order to perform an event-related analysis of epileptiform activity. Spikes are typically identified manually by an experienced observer, although methods for automatic spike detection have been proposed (Abd El-Samie et al., 2018).

Once spikes have been found within the data, it is then necessary to estimate the location of their source. Because the aim is to detect a single, focal area of cortex that acts as the epileptogenic zone, it is often assumed that the source of each spike should correspond to a single equivalent current dipole, and therefore dipole fitting is the most frequently used method to identify the location of the source. The best fitting single dipole is found for each spike and the consistency of the location of this dipole can then be compared across spikes.

Figure 5.10 shows an example of the location (and orientation) of dipoles fit to epileptiform spikes for three example patients, taken from the work of Oishsi and colleagues (Oishi et al., 2006). Each circle corresponds to the location of a dipole fit to an individual spike, while the line extending from the circle indicates the dipole orientation. Where the dipoles show a high degree of consistency in their location and orientation (such as for patient A in Figure 5.10) then this supports the presence of a single epileptogenic zone that might be effectively removed with a focal resection of cortical tissue. By contrast, where the dipole locations and orientations show a wide

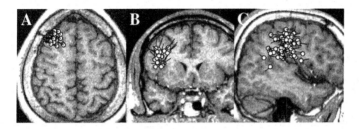

Figure 5.10 Location and orientation of dipole fits to epileptiform spikes in three epilepsy patients (labelled A, B & C) who underwent pre-surgical evaluation. *Reprinted from Oishi et al. (2006) Single and multiple clusters of magnetoencephalographic dipoles in neocortical epilepsy: Significance in characterizing the epileptogenic zone, Epilepsia, © 2006 International League Against Epilepsy.*

dispersion (such as for patient C in Figure 5.10) or the dipoles are localised to two or more discrete areas of cortex, this may tend to suggest the need for a more extensive surgical resection or of the need to resect multiple areas of cortex. Surgery is less likely to be successful in preventing seizures when this is the case.

A secondary role for MEG in pre-surgical evaluation is in pre-surgical functional mapping. When determining which areas of cortex to remove it is important for surgeons to avoid resecting what is known as *eloquent cortex*, that is the parts of cortex that are responsible for critical brain functions such as language and motor control. Thus, prior to surgery, it is important to determine the functional role of any area of cortex that is due to be removed. Source localisation of MEG event-related responses can play a role in this process: for instance, measurement of event-related responses occurring during a language task can be used to identify regions of the cortex involved in language processing that should be avoided during surgery. In general, the methods used for pre-surgical mapping of event-related responses are the same as those described in Section 5.1, so we will not present them in further detail here (see Kreidenhuber, De Tiège, & Rampp (2019) for a review of these methods).

5.3.2 Summary

MEG is not purely a research method but can also be used in clinical assessment. Currently the main clinical use of MEG is in pre-surgical evaluation in epilepsy. In some drug resistant forms of epilepsy, surgical resection of an area of cortex that causes the epilepsy – known as the epileptogenic zone – can be an effective treatment. Source localisation of epileptic discharges measured with MEG can be used to help identify the location of the epileptogenic zone and help to guide surgery (as well as helping to predict the likelihood that surgery will be successful). Measurement of event-related responses using MEG can also play a role in pre-surgical mapping of the location of areas of cortex responsible for critical brain functions that should be avoided during surgery.

5.4 Concluding remarks

Over the last 30 years, magnetoencephalography has developed from a niche methodology practised in a small number of specialist labs to a more widely used tool in human neuroscience. With the recent introduction of OPM-MEG it is likely the technique will become even more widely used over the next 30 years. Although there are a wide range of articles covering the technical aspects of MEG instrumentation and data analysis, there are still relatively few resources that provide a non-technical introduction to MEG. Hopefully, this book serves – at least in part – to fill that gap.

By necessity the book has only been able to give a general introduction to working with MEG. The technique offers a rich source of data on brain activity and, while the chapters on analysis and applications introduce some of the ways that MEG can be used, the range of methods and uses for MEG are far beyond what a short book like this can cover. At the end of each chapter a selection of further reading has been suggested. If you plan to become a regular user of MEG then you will greatly benefit from reading these suggested texts, as well as performing your own literature search on areas of most interest to you.

Good luck in your future endeavours with MEG!

Further reading

Bastos, A. M., & Schoffelen, J-M. (2016). A tutorial review of functional connectivity analysis methods and their interpretational pitfalls. *Frontiers in Systems Neuroscience, 9*, 175. https://doi.org/10.3389/fnsys.2015.00175

Brookes M.J., Woolrich M.W., & Price D. (2014) An introduction to MEG connectivity measurements. In Supek S., & Aine C. (Eds.) *Magnetoencephalography: From Signals to Dynamic Cortical Networks*, 321–358. Springer. https://doi.org/10.1007/978-3-642-33045-2_16

Gross, J. (2019). Magnetoencephalography in cognitive neuroscience: a primer. *Neuron, 104*(2), 189–204. https://doi.org/10.1016/j.neuron.2019.07.001

Hari, R., & Salmelin, R. (2011). Magnetoencephalography: From SQUIDs to neuroscience. *NeuroImage, 61*(2), 386–396. https://doi.org/10.1016/j.neuroimage.2011.11.074

Hari, R. et al. (2018). IFCN-endorsed practical guidelines for clinical magnetoencephalography (MEG), *Clinical Neurophysiology, 129*(8), 1720–1747. https://doi.org/10.1016/j.clinph.2018.03.042

Uhlhaas P. J., Liddle P., Linden D. E. J, Nobre A. C., Singh K. D., & Gross J. (2017). Magnetoencephalography as a tool in psychiatric research: Current status and perspective. *Biological Psychiatry: Cognitive Neuroscience and Neuroimaging, 2*(3), 235–244. https://doi.org/10.1016/j.bpsc.2017.01.005

References

Abd El-Samie, F. E., Alotaiby, T. N., Khalid, M. I., Alshebeili, S. A., & Aldosari, S. A. (2018). A review of EEG and MEG epileptic spike detection algorithms. *IEEE Access, 6*, 60673–60688. https://doi.org/10.1109/ACCESS.2018.2875487

Berger, H. (1929). Über das elektrenkephalogramm des menschen. *Archiv Für Psychiatrie Und Nervenkrankheiten, 87*(1). https://doi.org/10.1007/BF01797193

Biswal, B., Zerrin Yetkin, F., Haughton, V. M., & Hyde, J. S. (1995). Functional connectivity in the motor cortex of resting human brain using echo-planar MRI. *Magnetic Resonance in Medicine, 34*(4), 537–541. https://doi.org/10.1002/MRM.1910340409

Brookes, M. J., Woolrich, M., Luckhoo, H., Price, D., Hale, J. R., Stephenson, M. C., Barnes, G. R., Smith, S. M., & Morris, P. G. (2011). Investigating the electrophysiological basis of resting state networks using magnetoencephalography. *Proceedings of the National Academy of Sciences of the United States of America, 108*(40), 16783–16788. https://doi.org/ 10.1073/pnas.1112685108

de Cheveigné, A., & Nelken, I. (2019). Filters: When, why, and how (not) to use them. *Neuron, 102*(2), 280–293. https://doi.org/10.1016/J.NEU RON.2019.02.039

Deffke, I., Sander, T., Heidenreich, J., Sommer, W., Curio, G., Trahms, L., & Lueschow, A. (2007). MEG/EEG sources of the 170-ms response to faces are co-localized in the fusiform gyrus. *NeuroImage, 35*(4), 1495–1501. https://doi.org/10.1016/j.neuroimage.2007.01.034

Engels, M. M. A., Yu, M., Stam, C. J., Gouw, A. A., van der Flier, W. M., Scheltens, P., van Straaten, E. C. W., & Hillebrand, A. (2017). Directional information flow in patients with Alzheimer's disease. A source-space resting-state MEG study. *NeuroImage: Clinical, 15*(June), 673–681. https:// doi.org/10.1016/j.nicl.2017.06.025

Haegens, S., Händel, B. F., & Jensen, O. (2011). Top-down controlled alpha band activity in somatosensory areas determines behavioral perform- ance in a discrimination task. *Journal of Neuroscience, 31*(14), 5197–5204. https://doi.org/10.1523/JNEUROSCI.5199-10.2011

Halgren, E., Dhond, R. P., Christensen, N., Van Petten, C., Marinkovic, K., Lewine, J. D., & Dale, A. M. (2002). N400-like magnetoencephalography responses modulated by semantic context, word frequency, and lex- ical class in sentences. *NeuroImage, 17*(3), 1101–1116. https://doi.org/ 10.1006/nimg.2002.1268

Hamandi, K., Singh, K. D., & Muthukumaraswamy, S. (2011). Reduced movement-related beta desynchronisation in juvenile myoclonic epi- lepsy: A MEG study of task specific cortical modulation. *Clinical Neurophysiology, 122*(11), 2128–2138. https://doi.org/10.1016/J.CLI NPH.2011.04.017

Hipp, J. F., Hawellek, D. J., Corbetta, M., Siegel, M., & Engel, A. K. (2012). Large-scale cortical correlation structure of spontaneous oscillatory activity. *Nature Neuroscience, 15*(6), 884–890. https://doi.org/10.1038/ nn.3101

Jurkiewicz, M. T., Gaetz, W. C., Bostan, A. C., & Cheyne, D. (2006). Post- movement beta rebound is generated in motor cortex: Evidence from neuromagnetic recordings. *NeuroImage, 32*(3), 1281–1289. https://doi. org/10.1016/j.neuroimage.2006.06.005

Kanwisher, N., & Yovel, G. (2006). The fusiform face area: A cortical region specialized for the perception of faces. *Philosophical Transactions of the Royal Society B: Biological Sciences, 361*(1476), 2109–2128. https://doi.org/ 10.1098/rstb.2006.1934

Kiebel, S. J., Garrido, M. I., Moran, R. J., & Friston, K. J. (2008). Dynamic causal modelling for EEG and MEG. *Cognitive Neurodynamics, 2*(2), 121. https://doi.org/10.1007/S11571-008-9038-0

Koelewijn, L., Bompas, A., Tales, A., Brookes, M. J., Muthukumaraswamy, S. D., Bayer, A., & Singh, K. D. (2017). Alzheimer's disease disrupts alpha and beta-band resting-state oscillatory network connectivity. *Clinical Neurophysiology, 128*(11), 2347–2357. https://doi.org/10.1016/J.CLINPH.2017.04.018

Koelewijn, L., Hamandi, K., Brindley, L. M., Brookes, M. J., Routley, B. C., Muthukumaraswamy, S. D., Williams, N., Thomas, M. A., Kirby, A., te Water Naudé, J., Gibbon, F., & Singh, K. D. (2015). Resting-state oscillatory dynamics in sensorimotor cortex in benign epilepsy with centrotemporal spikes and typical brain development. *Human Brain Mapping, 36*(10), 3935–3949. https://doi.org/10.1002/hbm.22888

Kreidenhuber, R., De Tiège, X., & Rampp, S. (2019). Presurgical functional cortical mapping using electromagnetic source imaging. *Frontiers in Neurology, 10*(June), 1–14. https://doi.org/10.3389/fneur.2019.00628

Nolte, G., Bai, O., Wheaton, L., Mari, Z., Vorbach, S., & Hallett, M. (2004). Identifying true brain interaction from EEG data using the imaginary part of coherency. *Clinical Neurophysiology, 115*(10). https://doi.org/10.1016/j.clinph.2004.04.029

Nugent, A. C., Robinson, S. E., Coppola, R., Furey, M. L., & Zarate, C. A. (2015). Group differences in MEG-ICA derived resting state networks: Application to major depressive disorder. *NeuroImage, 118*. https://doi.org/10.1016/j.neuroimage.2015.05.051

Oishi, M., Kameyama, S., Masuda, H., Tohyama, J., Kanazawa, O., Sasagawa, M., & Otsubo, H. (2006). Single and multiple clusters of magnetoencephalographic dipoles in neocortical epilepsy: Significance in characterizing the epileptogenic zone. *Epilepsia, 47*(2), 355–364. https://doi.org/10.1111/j.1528-1167.2006.00428.x

Shahin, A., Roberts, L. E., Pantev, C., Trainor, L. J., & Ross, B. (2005). Modulation of P2 auditory-evoked responses by the spectral complexity of musical sounds. *NeuroReport, 16*(16), 1781–1785. https://doi.org/10.1097/01.wnr.0000185017.29316.63

Stam, C. J., Nolte, G., & Daffertshofer, A. (2007). Phase lag index: Assessment of functional connectivity from multi channel EEG and MEG with diminished bias from common sources. *Human Brain Mapping, 28*(11), 1178–1193. https://doi.org/10.1002/hbm.20346

Stefan, H., & Rampp, S. (2020). Interictal and Ictal MEG in presurgical evaluation for epilepsy surgery. *Acta Epileptologica 2020–2:1, 2*(1), 1–10. https://doi.org/10.1186/S42494-020-00020-2

van Diessen, E., Numan, T., van Dellen, E., van der Kooi, A. W., Boersma, M., Hofman, D., van Lutterveld, R., van Dijk, B. W., van Straaten, E. C. W., Hillebrand, A., & Stam, C. J. (2015). Opportunities and methodological challenges in EEG and MEG resting state functional brain network research. *Clinical Neurophysiology*, *126*(8), 1468–1481. https://doi.org/10.1016/j.clinph.2014.11.018

Glossary

Aliasing. An effect in which signals at different frequencies may produce identical data after sampling. In the context of MEG data acquisition, where the magnetic field measurements contain signals at frequencies above the Nyquist frequency this leads to signals incorrectly appearing at corresponding frequencies below the Nyquist frequency after sampling. To prevent this problem the signal is generally passed through an anti-aliasing filter prior to digitisation.

Artefact. A general term for any signal present in MEG data that does not reflect signal originating in the brain. This can include physiological artefacts (such as those due to head movements, eye blinks, etc.) and artefacts originating in the surrounding environment (such as those due to ferromagnetic materials or electromagnetic interference from lab equipment).

Baseline correction. A correction performed on MEG time series data by subtracting the mean amplitude offset within a baseline time interval from all data within an epoch (or from all data within the average time series). This ensures that the amplitude of event-related responses is measured relative to zero. When working in the frequency and time–frequency domains baseline correction may additionally (or alternatively) take the form of subtraction of the baseline spectral power from the spectrum of the event-related response.

Beamforming. An approach to MEG source analysis that uses spatial filtering to estimate source currents at locations of interest in the brain. This can be applied over a grid of locations across the brain volume to produce an image of source activity or can be used to estimate the source timeseries at individual locations (the latter is known as *virtual sensor* or *virtual electrode* analysis).

Block design. An experimental design structured so that different conditions are separated into blocks, and brain signals are quantified by averaging data across blocks of the same condition rather than across a series of individual events (see **event-related design**). Alternatively known as a *boxcar design*.

Cluster-based analysis. An approach to statistical analysis of MEG data based on identifying clusters of contiguous samples showing an experimental effect of interest and performing statistical testing on properties of those clusters. Because statistical testing is not performed separately at each sample this avoids the need for correction for multiple comparisons but has the disadvantage that statistical effects cannot be localised to any individual samples.

Complex number. A number that has a real and imaginary part. Data can be represented in the frequency and time–frequency domain by a single complex number (rather than two vales corresponding to magnitude and phase). Some forms of mathematical analysis can be performed more simply when the data is represented in this way.

Coregistration. The process of spatial aligning the subject's MRI to their MEG data. This is a necessary step for generating a head model in order to perform source analysis. Coregistration is usually performed by matching the MRI head surface with a digital representation of the subject's head surface collected during the MEG data acquisition.

Cross-frequency coupling. The phenomenon in which measurements of signals at two different frequencies show some consistent relationship. This most commonly takes the form of phase-amplitude coupling, where the amplitude of one frequency varies with the phase of a lower frequency, but other forms of coupling (such as phase-phase and amplitude-amplitude coupling) may also occur.

Current dipole. A theoretical current of infinitesimal length. When performing source estimation, one or more current dipoles are generally used to model the impressed currents that act as sources of the brain's magnetic field.

Dipole fitting. A method of source estimation performed by fitting the magnetic field expected from one or more dipolar sources to the measured data. This method works most effectively when the magnetic field can be explained by a small number of focal sources.

Dipole moment. Magnitude of the current represented by a current dipole, typically measured in units of ampere-metre [Am].

Envelope. The timeseries of instantaneous magnitude of a signal whose amplitude varies over time. This can be measured from the time–frequency representation of the data, or directly from the time domain representation of the data using a mathematical technique known as *the Hilbert transform*.

Epoch. A segment of data extracted from a time interval within the MEG data timeseries. Typically selected so that the data within the epoch is time-locked to an experimental event of interest.

Event-related design. An experimental design that is structured around a series of experimental events (such as the presentation of stimuli). This is the most common experimental design used with MEG.

Event-related field (ERF). A change in the amplitude of the magnetic field time-locked to an experimental event and typically measured by averaging data across epochs in the time domain. A comparable response – the *event-related potential* – can measured with EEG.

Evoked response. A brain response that is reflected in a change in amplitude that is time-locked (and phase-locked in the case of periodic responses) to an experimental event and therefore can be measured by averaging data in the time domain across epochs that are also time-locked to the corresponding event.

False discovery rate (FDR). A measure of the rate of type I errors that can be used as a criterion for statistical significance where it is necessary to correct for multiple statistical comparisons. The rate defines the expected proportion of significant results across the group of tests that correspond to type I errors.

Familywise error rate (FWER). A measure of the expected probability of finding at least one type I error across a group of statistical tests. Controlling for this rate is one method of correction for multiple statistical comparisons.

Field spread. The phenomenon whereby the magnetic field from an individual source current spreads across multiple sensors on the sensor array. This limits the precision at which brain responses can be localised in sensor space as well as falsely inflating the degree of functional connectivity between sensors that are close together.

Forward model. A mathematical model that predicts the magnetic field measured at the sensors for a given source current in the brain. This is calculated from a source model (usually a current dipole) that predicts the magnetic field generated by the impressed current and a head model that predicts the magnetic field generated by the volume current. The creation of a forward model is necessary for performing source estimation.

Fourier transform. A mathematical transform that converts a data time series into a series of measurements of magnitude and phase (or their complex-valued equivalent) across frequencies.

Frequency domain. Representation of MEG data for processing and analysis as a series of measurements over frequency. Data can be transformed from the time domain to the frequency domain using the Fourier transform.

Frequency spectrum. A visual representation of frequency domain data in which signal measures (such as amplitude or power) are plotted against frequency. See also **power spectrum**.

Functional connectivity. Measure of brain connectivity based on the extent to which activity in one brain area influences activity in another area. This is quantified by measuring the presence of statistical relationships between the time series of two or more sensors or sources. Many such statistical relationships can be measured from MEG data time series, and therefore there are multiple methods for quantifying functional connectivity from MEG data.

Gradiometer. A magnetic field sensor that measures the difference in the strength of the magnetic field between two pick-up coils. If the distance between the coils is known, then this gives the gradient of the magnetic field. MEG gradiometers come in two spatial configurations: axial (which measure the field gradient in a direction perpendicular to the surface of the MEG helmet) and planar (which measure the field gradient in a direction parallel to the surface of the MEG helmet).

Head localisation coils. Small coils that are attached to the head during MEG data acquisition in order to measure the position of the subject's head relative to the MEG helmet. This can be used to monitor the participant's head movements during data acquisition. Information about the subject's head position within the MEG helmet is also necessary to perform coregistration of the subjects MRI with their MEG data. Also known as **head position indicator coils**.

Head model. A mathematical model of the subject's head that is used to estimate the magnetic field generated by the volume currents as part of the forward model. An accurate head model must precisely model the shape and conductive properties of each of the head tissues, but good approximations can be achieved using simplifying assumptions, such as that the head is formed from spherical volumes.

Impressed current. The name given to current flow within neurons generated by postsynaptic potentials which, along with volume/secondary currents, generate the brain's magnetic field. It is the distribution of impressed current that is estimated when performing source analysis. Also known as **primary current**.

Independent component analysis. A method for decomposing data into multiple statistically independent components. In MEG data analysis is this is commonly used as a method for separating and removing artefacts from the data.

Induced response. A brain response that is reflected in a change in signal power time-locked to an experimental event, but where signal phase is not locked to the event, meaning that the data cannot be measured by averaging data across epochs in the time domain. Instead, induced responses must be measured by averaging amplitude or power in the frequency or time–frequency domains.

Inverse problem. The problem of estimating a model from a set of physical measurements. In the context of MEG, this corresponds to the problem of estimating the sources currents present in the brain from the magnetic field measurements. The MEG inverse problem is ill-posed, because for any given magnetic field measurements there are multiple source distributions that could fit the data, and no unique solution can be found from the data alone. Thus, to perform MEG source estimation additional constraints must be imposed to find a unique solution to the inverse problem.

Latency. A measure of the timing of brain responses relative to the timing of an experimental event.

Lead field. A matrix (or set of matrices) that give the relationship between a source of unit moment at each location (and orientation) in source space and the predicted magnetic field generated by that source at each sensor. The lead field matrix is the most common way to represent the forward model when performing the calculations involved in MEG source estimation.

Magnetically shielded room. A room which has passive (and in some cases active) shielding of the exterior magnetic field. Generally, MEG systems are sited in a shielded room in order to reduce magnetic interference from the external environment.

Magnetometer. A sensor that measures the strength of the magnetic field at a given location (and direction). Along with gradiometers these form one of the two types of MEG sensor.

Mass univariate. A statistical analysis where the data at each sample are treated as a separate variable and statistical analysis is performed simultaneously across each of these variables.

Minimum norm estimation. An approach to MEG distributed source estimation in which the dipole moment is estimated simultaneously at all locations across the cortical surface (or within the cortical volume) subject to the constraint that the source estimate must correspond to the best fitting source distribution with the minimum source power. This constraint ensures that a unique solution to the MEG inverse problem can be achieved.

Multitapering. An approach to tapering data in the time domain prior to transforming into the frequency and time-frequency domains. Unlike conventional tapering when a single taper is applied, in multitapering several tapers are applied, and the result is averaged. This introduces greater smoothing in the frequency spectrum (or the spectrogram) of the data.

Nyquist frequency. The frequency equal to half the sampling rate. Signals at frequencies above the Nyquist frequency are aliased to corresponding frequencies below the Nyquist frequency (see **aliasing**).

Optically pumped magnetometer (OPM). A type of magnetic sensor recently introduced for use with MEG. Unlike SQUID-based sensors they do not require cooling to achieve superconductivity and therefore can mounted on the subject's head rather than placed inside a fixed helmet.

Phase. An angular quantity that represents the shift of a periodic signal along the time axis. Can also refer to instantaneous phase which measures where a periodic signal is in its cycle at a given time sample.

Phase coherence. A measure of the consistency of signal phase across epochs. This can be used to determine the extent a brain response is phase locked to an experimental event. Alternatively, may be used to measure functional connectivity between two sensors or sources by quantifying the consistency of the differences in phase between the two time series across epochs.

Power spectrum. A visual representation of the magnitude of the data in the frequency domain in which signal power is plotted against frequency.

Preprocessing. One or more processing steps used to format and clean the data prior to analysis. This can include segmenting the data into epcohs, applying temporal filtering and/or using one or more of the various methods for removing data aretfacts.

Primary current. See **impressed current**.

Radial (orientation). Within a spherical coordinate system (such as in a spherical head model) the radial orientation at any point within the sphere is the orientation away from or towards the centre of the sphere. Assuming a spherical head model, MEG is insensitive to source currents with a radial orientation.

Right-hand rule. A method for remembering the relationship between a current and the induced magnetic field. With the right-hand formed into a fist with the thumb upright, the magnetic field flows in the direction of the fingers (clockwise when viewed from below) when the current flows in the direction of the thumb.

Sampling rate. The rate (measured in Hertz) at which the continuous magnetic field measurements are converted into digital samples. This determines the temporal resolution of the MEG data. Sometimes alternatively known as *sampling frequency*.

Secondary current. See **volume current**.

Sensor space. Representation of the MEG data with respect to the spatial distribution of the magnetic field across sensors (as opposed to the spatial distribution across sources; see *source space*).

Signal-space projection. A method for removing data artefacts from MEG data, based on the assumption that brain and noise signals should have different spatial distributions across sensors. The spatial distribution of the noise signals is estimated from a data acquisition that contains only those signals (e.g. an empty room recording).

Signal-space separation. A method for separating MEG data into components that originate inside and outside of the MEG helmet based on knowledge of the exact geometry of the sensor array. This can be used as a method for removing data artefacts that originate outside of the MEG helmet.

Signal leakage. The phenomenon whereby signals generated from an individual source within the brain may leak into the estimates of other sources that share similar lead fields. This limits the extent to which brain signals can be localised to specific sources within the brain as well as falsely inflating the degree of functional connectivity between sources that are close together. Alternatively know as **source leakage**.

Source estimation. The process of estimating the underlying source currents in the brain that gave rase to a magnetic field measured with MEG. There are many different methods for achieving this, with no single method guaranteed to be accurate in all circumstances due to the ill-posed nature of the MEG inverse problem. Sometimes alternatively know as **source reconstruction** or **source localisation**.

Source leakage. See **signal leakage**.

Source model. Mathematical model of source currents in the brain. This model is used to calculate the magnetic field produced by impressed current at a given location and orientation as part of the calculation of the MEG forward model. This model is generally a *current dipole*.

Source space. Representation of the MEG data with respect to the spatial distribution of estimated sources of the magnetic field.

Spectral leakage. A phenomenon in which signal at a specific frequency is leaked to other frequencies within the spectrum of the data. This occurs when periodic signals fit within the measurement interval (such an epoch) a non-integer number of times and can be reduced by applying some form of *tapering* to the data.

Spectrogram. A visual representation of data in the time-frequency domain. Spectrograms are typically plotted with time on the x-axis and frequency on the y-axis. Signal measurements (e.g. amplitude or power) at each time–frequency sample are represented at the corresponding point on the plot by mapping their value to a colour.

Superconducting QUantum Interference Device (SQUID). A type of magnetic sensor that is currently the most frequently used for acquiring MEG measurements. SQUIDs rely on the property of *superconductivity* to work and therefore must be cooled to –269°C. SQUID-based sensors can be configured to operate as *magnetometers* or *gradiometers*.

Tangential (orientation). Within a spherical coordinate system (such as in a spherical head model) the tangential orientations at any point within the sphere are the orientations that are at right-angles to the radial orientation (see **radial (orientation)**). Assuming a spherical head model, MEG is must sensitive to source currents with a tangential orientation.

Tapering. A process of multiplying a data time series with a taper function (i.e. a function that is maximal at the centre and decreases towards the edges) prior to transformation into the frequency or time-frequency domains. This reduces *spectral leakage* but also smooths the frequency spectrum, reducing the frequency resolution of the data.

Temporal filtering. A form of signal processing applied to data time series that attenuates signals at specific frequencies while allowing signal at other frequencies to pass unaffected. Filters can be designed to pass frequencies either above (*high-pass* filtering) or below (*low-pass* filtering) a cut-off frequency. Alternatively, filters can pass (*band-pass* filtering) or attenuate (*band-stop* filtering) signals between a pair of cut-off frequencies.

Time domain. Representation of MEG data for processing and analysis as a series of measurements over time.

Time–frequency domain. Representation of MEG data for processing and analysis as a series of measurements over time and frequency. Data can be transformed from the time domain to the time-frequency domain using transforms such as the short-time Fourier transform and the wavelet transform.

Trigger. A signal sent from the stimulus computer or from experimental hardware (e.g. a response device) and recorded in the MEG data to signal the timing of an experimental event within the data acquisition. This is necessary in order to analyse MEG data relative to experimental events.

Type I error. In statistical testing a type I error (also known as a *false positive*) refers to the situation in which the null hypothesis is rejected despite being true. In statistical testing involving MEG data there are usually multiple simultaneous tests and therefore it is typical to control for the type I error rate across the family of tests using measures such as the familywise error rate or the false discovery rate.

Type II error. In statistical testing a type II error (also known as a *false negative*) refers to the situation in which the null hypothesis is not rejected despite being false. The type II error rate determines the statistical power of tests to detect experimental effects. Because statistical testing of MEG data often involves some form of correction for multiple comparisons that tends to increase the type II error rate, it is generally important to ensure that the tests still have sufficient power to detect experimental effects of interest.

Volume current. The name given to current flowing within the brain volume due to impressed currents occurring within neurons. The magnetic fields generated by volume currents contribute to the MEG measurements and therefore must be accounted for in the forward model wh en performing source estimation. This is achieved by using the head model to model the flow of current (and the corresponding magnetic field) through the head volume. Also known as **secondary current**.

Index

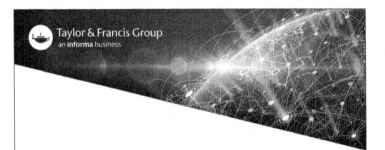